Fitness, Technology and Society

The fitness industry is experiencing a new boom characterized by the proliferation of interactive and customizable technology, from exercise-themed video games to smartphone apps to wearable fitness trackers. This new technology presents the possibility of boundless self-tracking, generating highly personalized data for self-assessment and for sharing among friends. While this may be beneficial – for example, in encouraging physical activity – the new fitness boom also raises important questions about the very nature of our relationship with technology. This is the first book to examine these questions through a critical scholarly lens.

Addressing key themes such as consumer experience, gamification, and surveillance, *Fitness, Technology and Society: Amusing Ourselves to Life* argues that fitness technologies, by 'datafying' the body and daily experience, are turning fitness into a constant pursuit. The book explores the origins of contemporary fitness technologies, considers their implications for consumers, producers, and society in general, and reflects on what they suggest about the future of fitness experience.

Casting new light on theories of society, technology, and the body, this is fascinating reading for all those interested in technology, physical cultural studies, and the sociology of sport.

Brad Millington is a Lecturer (Assistant Professor) in the Department for Health at the University of Bath, United Kingdom. Previously, he completed a PhD in Kinesiology at the University of British Columbia and held a Postdoctoral Fellowship at the University of Toronto. His research is broadly focused on physical culture and the meanings, practices, and technologies associated with the active body. In 2016, he was the recipient of the Sociology of Sport Journal Early Career Researcher Award.

Routledge Research in Sport, Culture and Society

For a full list of titles in this series, please visit www.routledge.com/sport/series/RRSCS

Fitness, Technology and Society

Amusing Ourselves to Life

Brad Millington

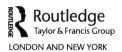

Routledge
Taylor & Francis Group

LONDON AND NEW YORK

First published 2018
by Routledge
2 Park Square, Milton Park, Abingdon, Oxon OX14 4RN

and by Routledge
711 Third Avenue, New York, NY 10017

Routledge is an imprint of the Taylor & Francis Group, an informa business

© 2018 Brad Millington

British Library Cataloguing-in-Publication Data
A catalogue record for this book is available from the British Library

Library of Congress Cataloging-in-Publication Data
A catalog record for this book has been requested

ISBN: 978-1-138-94803-7 (hbk)
ISBN: 978-1-315-66974-8 (ebk)

Typeset in Sabon
by Apex CoVantage, LLC

Contents

Preface

It's January. I am lying in bed with my partner. Both of us are reading on our phones, as modern couples do.

"Look at this," she says. "Look how little we walked over the holidays." She turns her phone to me. There's a line chart bobbing up and down showing steps taken on a monthly basis. The line takes a sharp dive in December. It's yet to recover.

"You track your steps on your phone?" I ask. "No. Well, yes. I guess. This is my new phone. I guess the app was running, but I didn't know it."

"We do drive a lot over the holidays when we're with our families," I say. She responds, like me, looking for a rationale: "Yeah. And it's *the holidays*."

"Let's go for a long walk this weekend," she says.

"Funny that it was tracking you without you knowing."

* * * * *

Such is the promise of contemporary fitness technologies. Tracking generates data, which generates insight, which generates behaviour change – and maybe a dose of shame. That data can be produced and perhaps shared without our knowledge is just part of the process.

Acknowledgements

Chapter 2 of this book is derived in part from an article published in *Leisure Studies* on 4 December 2014, available online: http://www.tandfonline.com/ doi/10.1080/02614367.2014.986511. Millington, B. (2016). Video games and the political and cultural economies of health-entertainment. *Leisure Studies*, 35(6), 739–757.

Chapter 5 is derived in part from Millington, B. (2015). Exergaming in retirement centres and the integration of media and physical literacies. *Journal of Aging Studies*, 35, 160–168. DOI: http://doi.org/10.1016/j.jaging. 2015.08.005.

The Chapter 3 and the conclusion chapter are derived in part from Millington, B., Fit for prosumption: Interactivity and the second fitness boom, Media, Culture & Society (38.8) pp. 1184–1200. Copyright © 2016, Brad Millington. Reprinted by permission of Sage Publications. https://doi. org/10.1177/0163443716643150.

Chapter 5 is based in part on research funded by a Social Sciences and Humanities Research Council of Canada Postdoctoral Fellowship and a Sport Canada Sport Participation Research Initiative award.

* * * * *

This book is owed to the generosity, wisdom, and support of many people.

Thank you to my friends, colleagues, and students at the University of Bath, University of Toronto, The University of British Columbia, Queen's University, and in the academic community in general; Brian Wilson, Patricia Vertinsky, and Margaret MacNeill; Simon Whitmore, William Bailey, Cecily Davey, and everyone involved in the review and production processes; my friends and family in the United Kingdom, Toronto, Vancouver, Kingston, Ottawa, and beyond; the Anderton group; Mom, Dad, Rob, Scott, Suneeta, Jaya, Kiran, and Bodhi; and, of course, Katie and Theo, who know all my favourite chords.

Introduction

The new fitness boom

The cover art for Neil Postman's (1986) book *Amusing Ourselves to Death* presents one of the more evocative images in the history of technology criticism. A meticulously presented family sit together on a pink sofa: mother, father, daughter, and son. The mother wears a dress, cardigan, and pearl necklace. The father wears a buttoned shirt and sweater. The son and daughter are well outfitted too. In the foreground, facing the family, sits a television set, its light shining onto parents and children both. A silhouette is cast on the back wall. All is normal, save for the family's missing heads.

Fast-forward twenty years to the mid-2000s and the images accompanying the release of the Nintendo Wii – a gaming console from the world's most successful video game maker – could hardly be any more different. Still facing a TV set, the protagonists in Nintendo's promotional materials were in many cases uprooted from the living room sofa, not confined to it like the headless family of *Amusing Ourselves to Death*. One early advertising campaign for the Wii showed two businessmen – presumably Nintendo employees – appearing on people's doorsteps with a console and a request: "We [Wii] would like to play" (Jones & Thiruvathukal, 2012, p. 140). On their first stop in one advertisement, the businessmen encounter a mother, father, son, and daughter, who before long are mimicking sporting gestures as they engage with games like Wii Bowling and Wii Tennis. The Wii, after all, rests on an active style of play whereby a motion-capturing remote controller allows 'real' movement to be replicated on-screen. Far from a space of imminent death, the living room thus becomes a setting for liveliness – for *life* – courtesy a new form of human-technology interactivity. Heads were fully in tact across Nintendo's advertising campaign.

* * * * *

The argument at the heart of this book is that we are in the midst of a new fitness boom – one characterized by the proliferation of interactive and highly personalized health and fitness technologies. The language of a 'fitness boom' likely rings familiar. The 1970s and 1980s were a time when fitness allegedly 'boomed' as well. As explored in detail in Chapter 1 herein, exercise fads emerged on the scene at this time, often replete with their own unique cultures and aesthetics, aerobics being the most notable case in point. Already-established activities grew more popular too. The 1970s saw the onset of a 'running craze', for example, whereby marathoners and weekend warriors alike took to the streets in pursuit of better health (Latham, 2015; Radar, 1991; Scheerder, Breedveld, & Borgers, 2015). Purveyors of fitness apparel reaped the rewards of this growing interest in fitness in a financial sense. The 1980s were the decade that Nike transitioned from a shoe company to an iconic, global brand, facing competition from adidas and Reebok (among others) in the process, and using a strategy of appealing directly to women as a way of expanding the company's market share. Fitness celebrities such as Jane Fonda implored their followers to set their sights on the rogue fatty tissue blemishing their bums, bellies, and thighs.

From the 1970s onwards, fitness was newly institutionalized as well in that fitness gyms – often fitted with the latest fitness technologies – saw an upsurge in interest. The home was (re)imagined as a fitness site too, once again through technological innovation in that electronic technologies like treadmills were marketed as tools for getting fit without leaving the house. Governments took an interest in fitness with the health and wellbeing of the population in mind. This was shown, for example, in the expansion of the Presidential Physical Fitness Awards under Richard Nixon's administration in the United States (U.S. Department of Health & Human Services, n.d.a). Initiatives of this kind were not pursued without evidence, as the promotion of activities like jogging was driven in part by a growing body of scientific evidence on the short- and long-term repercussions of sedentary living (Eisenman & Barnett, 1979; Latham, 2015). All told, and while the 'fitness boom' is no doubt a nebulous term, the 1970s and 1980s were a time when fitness clearly took on new dimensions and renewed importance.

The claim here, however, is that a *new* fitness boom is upon us – that something has changed. Certainly, fitness did not disappear at the end of the 1980s. What basis is there to claim that a new fitness boom has arrived?

In one sense, this is a new fitness boom in that the fitness *market* is evidently booming – as shown most of all by the sheer breadth of health and fitness technologies available for use, whether by intrepid or aspiring fitness enthusiasts. This is true especially when it comes to smartphone-compatible application software, or 'apps', available for download from online app stores. Estimates of the number of health and fitness apps available for download are difficult to find – an indicator, perhaps, of the overwhelming size of the app marketplace. One report from 2015 put the figure at over 165,000 mHealth (mobile health) apps in Apple and Android app stores (Terry, 2015; The Economist, 2016). As of February 2017, there are 21 web pages in the U.S. Apple app store listing names of health and fitness apps starting with the letter 'D' alone, with roughly 150 apps per page.

This is the "age of the app" (Lorinc, Tossell, & el Akkad, 2010). But perhaps even more significant than the sheer number of health and fitness apps available for download is the growth trajectory of products of this kind. In June 2014, the analytics company Flurry reported a 33% increase in mobile app usage in general to that point in the calendar year and a 62% increase in the usage of health and fitness apps specifically. The company Citrix's 2015 mobile analytics report noted that fitness apps in particular were dominating the wider health app category, with 78% of health app users engaging with apps devoted specifically to fitness (Citrix, 2015). Taken together, 'health and fitness' is now a standout category in a technology industry already noteworthy for its growing reach and influence. The fitness side of 'health and fitness' seems to be growing more prominent in particular, recognizing that the divide between health and fitness is somewhat unclear (see below). When the apparel company Under Armour acquired the apps MyFitnessPal and Endomondo – reportedly paying nearly half a billion dollars for the former (Mitroff, 2015) – it was a sign that health and fitness apps are worthy of both corporate and consumer attention.

The growth of the fitness market is owed to the growing prominence of *wearable* (and usually app-compatible) health and fitness technologies such as activity-tracking wristbands as well. Business is no doubt booming for Fitbit, for example – a fitness brand that, at the start of 2017, was reported to have sold over 54 million wearable devices from its expansive product catalogue and to have the most popular health and fitness app of all, judging at least by U.S. downloads (BusinessWire, 2017). With users such as former American president Barack Obama in tow, Fitbit's success comes in a marketplace crowded with rival brands, including competitors with the deepest of pockets. Through wristbands and smartwatches in particular, companies ranging from Microsoft to Garmin to Nike to the Chinese technology company Xiaomi and far beyond have all made their way into the health and fitness 'space' in recent years. Smart *clothing* has a health and fitness dimension too. Having acquired two prominent health and fitness apps, Under Armour's plan, per *Wired* magazine, is "to turn your clothes into gadgets" (Pierce, 2016) – for example, in the form of smart shoes that record data on exercise activity. In all, global revenues for mHealth are forecasted to reach $21.5 billion in 2018 (The Economist, 2016). By 2020, wearable tech alone is expected to be worth $34 billion (Lamkin, 2016).

Let us not forget Nintendo! A case will be made in Chapter 2 that Nintendo's release of its aforementioned Wii console in 2006 effectively marks the starting point of the new fitness boom. The Wii (re)launched the phenomenon known as exergaming, and, in the process, positioned interactive technologies as (arguably) valid tools in the quest for fit living. Going by Nintendo's own data, as of December 2016 the company had sold 101.63 million Wii units worldwide and 917.34 million software units to go along with this hardware. The fitness-themed titles Wii Fit and Wii Fit Plus are among

Nintendo's most successful games, each with more than 20 million units sold worldwide as of September 2016 (Nintendo, 2016). There is now a lengthy list of fitness-themed games compatible with either the Wii, Nintendo's successor consoles, or competitor devices made by rivals such as Sony and Microsoft – EA Sports Active, Jillian Michaels' Fitness Ultimatum, My Fitness Coach, and UFC Personal Trainer to name a few.

Thus, for many, fitness remains a profitable domain. Yet the claim that we are witnessing a new fitness boom is based not just on the proliferation of fitness technologies; it also stems from the idea that these technologies are helping to *fundamentally transform* the nature of fitness activity. This is a qualitative change in what is possible in fitness and not just a quantitative change in the range of technologies with which one could possibly engage.

What does this mean? As we shall see in Chapter 1, fitness luminaries have long urged that healthy living is an 'always-on' proposition – that daily activities ranging from sleeping to eating to exercise and beyond present the chance to 'know thyself' and, in the end, to make thyself better. The American strongman Charles Atlas reportedly went so far as to advocate for chewing milk, lest one miss out on the health benefits of regular mastication (Toon & Golden, 2002). Technologies such as dumbbells, weight pulleys, and, in the first fitness boom, electronic treadmills have served in the pursuit of fit living over time.

By contrast, the fitness technologies of the new fitness boom take knowing thyself to a new extent, and radically so. Take Fitbit's line of fitness technologies as a case in point. The Fitbit Surge, for example, is a 'super watch' that, like any watch, is made to accompany the user wherever she goes. The difference from a regular watch – or, indeed, a weight pulley or treadmill – is that the Surge device records performance metrics such as distance travelled, pace, elevation climbed, sleep, stationary time, and heart rate, all 'on the go' (Fitbit Inc., 2017). In turn, the device relays these measures to the Fitbit app so they can be represented on screen through features like maps of distance travelled and graphs showing heart rate changes during exercise. From the convergence of technology and flesh at the point of the wrist, the body is tracked, 'datafied', and represented – and thus potentially known to the technology user in new and productive ways. Indeed, the general idea in the new fitness boom is to draw highly personalized insights from technological enhancement. The idea too is to share these data widely, both intentionally via friend networks or online coaches and, perhaps unintentionally, with companies interested in the commodification of user data.

In the new fitness boom – let us call it Fitness 2.0 to allow for newer fitness booms down the road – fitness is 'always on' in that fitness technologies are ideally 'always on you' (see Turkle, 2008). The question remains: To what end? The new fitness boom, as we shall see, is in one sense about optimization, whether in the form of risk mitigation or simply making life better. Yet it is equally about having fun through 'gamified' experience. The politics of life meet the politics of amusement.

A tale of two discourses: the fitness boom and the obesity epidemic

Thus, the 'tools' at our disposable for getting fit are now highly sophisticated and abundant. The list of tools categorized under the letter 'D' alone is staggeringly long. What is noteworthy about Fitbit products and their kin, however, is not only their nature but also the context in which they have emerged. As our means for getting fit expand, we now encounter at the same time a ceaseless string of dire forecasts on the state of health and well-being at the population level. Said another way, we may well be in the midst of a new fitness boom, but we are equally in the midst of an alleged obesity epidemic.

Once again, this is not entirely new, meaning that dire forecasts on the state of the body politic have a lengthy history, as we shall see in the following chapter. Moreover, the obesity epidemic of the present moment is certainly contested terrain. From a critical biomedical perspective, it is effectively a function of poor science and over-generalization. From a libertarian perspective, obesity panic stands as an infringement on personal freedom to the extent that it restricts consumer options (e.g., via bans on unhealthy foods; see Lupton, 2012; Gard, 2011). Nonetheless, a functionalist, *anti*-obesity perspective reigns, certainly in the West, though the obesity epidemic is seen as an increasingly global phenomenon. Deborah Lupton (2012) describes the anti-obesity stance:

> Those researching and writing within the anti-obesity perspective – mainly including academics, policy makers, politicians and practitioners from within medicine, nutrition and public health areas such as epidemiology and health promotion, but also some researchers in the social sciences – tend to take an unproblematized approach to fat. For them, fatness – or what they prefer to term 'overweight' or 'obesity', or sometimes 'excess body weight' – is a major health risk for those who are designated as being overweight or obese, associated with such significant health problems as cardiovascular heart disease, diabetes and early death.
> (pp. 14–15)

Of course, the current moment is one of risk thinking in general. Health concerns extend far beyond obesity to matters such as pesticide exposure, water, and air quality, and beyond. But the obesity epidemic is the clearest representation of the idea that modern living is hindering *life itself*. Indeed, while obesity is generally deemed a precursor to illnesses such as diabetes and heart disease, it is equally seen as an *outcome* of precursor problems of other kinds. As one example, a recent Report of the Standing Senate Committee on Social Affairs, Science and Technology (2016) – a Canadian federal government report – sets out a macabre tone from the start: "There is an obesity crisis in this country. Canadians are paying for it with their wallets – and with their lives" (p. iv). It is said in turn that nearly two-thirds of adults and one-third of children are now either overweight or obese. Among other measures needed to 'tip the scales' towards a healthy future is the need for active living: "Canadians must renew their efforts to eat healthy and to get active – and government and industry must give citizens the means and motivation to make informed lifestyle choices" (Standing Senate Committee on Social Affairs, Science and Technology, 2016, p. iv). In Britain, obesity rhetoric recently took on an even starker tone when UK Chief Medical Officer Professor Dame Sally Davies warned that obesity in women was as dangerous as a terror threat (see Lay, 2015).

Against this backdrop, obesity and inactivity are often imagined as problems that require 'all hands on deck'. The scientific literature on obesity, for example, is attuned to the impact of 'obesogenic environments', such as contexts where healthy eating choices or physical activity options are absent or effectively inaccessible (e.g., see Lake, Townshend, & Alvanides, 2010). The aforementioned Standing Committee report is titled 'Obesity in Canada: A Whole of Society Approach for a Healthier Canada'. "From policy makers to parents," the report stresses, "industry insiders to family doctors, all Canadians have a role to play to beat back this crisis" (Standing Senate Committee on Social Affairs, Science and Technology, 2016, p. iv). This is not to discredit the view emanating from critical weight/obesity studies and fat studies that, in the time of an obesity crisis, "the emphasis is still overwhelmingly on the individual's responsibility" – and problematically so (Lupton, 2012, p. 41). Nor is the point to accept the premise that fat is the legible manifestation of underlying health problems without fail. This premise is generally rejected by critical scholars and fat activists as well. The point, instead, is that the obesity epidemic has helped instil the idea that contemporary life is poorly calibrated against our fundamental need for energy expenditure and for moderation in energy intake. The biopolitics of the present moment open up a 'space' for many actors interested in lifestyle change – people, companies, and 'things' among them.

What is especially compelling about the new fitness boom is not just that interactive health and fitness consumer technologies are now so prevalent, but that technology in general is shedding its reputation as a central force behind growing rates of inactivity. Certainly, this is no easy battle; screen time is still often correlated with inactivity (e.g., see ParticipACTION, 2016). But our screens are now positioned as our health and fitness allies as well. Through health and fitness apps, devices like smartphones and tablets become vessels for relaying alarming trends in (for example) one's Body Mass Index (a weight-to-height measure) or for connecting fitness participants to coaches and fitness trainers. The U.S. surgeon general's 2012 'Healthy Apps' Challenge, aimed at rewarding innovative apps that provide individually tailored health information and "empower the public to regularly engage in and enjoy health-promoting behaviors" (U.S. Department of Health & Human Services, n.d.b), symbolized the view that informa-tion and communication technologies (and their proprietors) are increas-ingly welcome in the fight against unhealthy living. The UK government's 2015 strategy for creating an active nation likewise shines a positive light on the technologies studied here. According to the report, fitness apps and wearable technology have made it possible to capture data and spur activ-ity; they will "define the world of sport and physical activity in the coming decade" (HM Government, 2015, p. 25). Chapter 2 of this book addresses the most remarkable case of technology 'bending back' towards healthy living – exergaming – and considers lessons that can be drawn from Nin-tendo's quest to reimagine video gaming as a healthy pastime for the family as a whole. In a time of crisis, it's 'all hands on deck', fitness and technology companies included.

Theorizing fitness

What is fitness? The question is, of course, important to any analysis of fitness and is one that can be answered from different disciplinary van-tage points. From a functional, biomedical perspective, fitness is associated with certain functional capacities. Fitness is, in one sense, a combination of strength, flexibility, and cardiovascular endurance; "it can be quantified and evaluated relative to established benchmarks" (Smith Maguire, 2008, p. 1). At the same time, measures of strength and endurance are sometimes con-nected to (functional) daily routines as well, as with the idea that physical fitness is, "the ability to carry out daily tasks with alertness and vigor, with-out undue fatigue, and with enough reserve to meet emergencies or to enjoy leisure time pursuits" (Glanze, 1986, p. 880; cited in Maud, 2006, p. 1). In this definition, fitness effectively stands as the 'physical' in the prevailing definition of health: "Health is a state of complete physical, mental and social well-being and not merely the absence of disease or infirmity" (World Health Organization, 2017). Physical *literacy* is a concept now associated with fitness as well (see Chapter 5). In 2010, Luc Tremblay and Meghann Lloyd described physical literacy as "the new kid on the block" (p. 26). They operationalized this concept by describing physical literacy's four constitu-ent components:

(a) physical fitness (cardio-respiratory, muscular strength and flex-ibility), (b) motor behaviour (fundamental motor skill proficiency), (c) physical activity behaviours (directly measured daily activity), and (d) psycho-social/cognitive factors (attitudes, knowledge, and feelings).
(p. 28)

For Tremblay and Lloyd (2010), physical literacy must be made measurable to be useful in contexts such as school-based physical education (PE) – for example, through tests of physical fitness. As Roberta Sassatelli (2010) writes in considering functionalist perspectives of this kind, fitness, as a concept, refers to both *training* and the *physical condition* that such training engenders.

By contrast, Jennifer Smith Maguire (2008) describes fitness as a cultural field, which is to say it is a site where fitness activity is ascribed meaning in different ways by different social actors, often in the interest of legitimizing a particular point of view. Fitness clubs, for example, tend to construe fitness as a commercial pursuit – one that can bestow physical capital in that a fit body has value (e.g., in seeking employment). Fitness media reinforce this definition while making fitness out to be a lifestyle tied to other forms of consumption (e.g., purchasing fitness apparel). Adding further complexity are lived definitions of fitness among people themselves, which tend to factor in matters such as societal norms and expectations – as promoted, for example, in advertising (Smith Maguire, 2008). These perspectives are, altogether, interrelated, each shining a different light on what fitness potentially means.

Yet perhaps the most compelling take on fitness, at least from a social sciences perspective, comes from Zygmunt Bauman's (2011) theorizing of 'liquid modernity' (also see Bauman, 1995). For Bauman, fitness is a concept with no upper limit – which is to say it is always pursuable, no matter one's already-existing fitness level. Indeed, it is this limitless quality that separates fitness from *health* in Bauman's account. Health has historically been seen as a relatively stable construct: "It refers to a bodily and psychical condition which allows the satisfaction of the demands of the socially designed and assigned role – and those demands tend to be constant and steady" (p. 77). This, at least, is how health is understood in producer societies; the 'designed and assigned' role involves one's role in the workforce. Fitness, by contrast, is anything but 'solid': "It cannot by its nature be pinned down and circumscribed with any precision" (Bauman, 2011, p. 77). Fitness in this regard is a concept for consumer societies. There is no end target for fitness; it is instead a state of constant self-scrutiny.

The supposed divide between health and fitness in Bauman's work may be unconvincing – and, indeed, his argument in part is that this divide is increasingly under erasure. Health is increasingly subject to fitness's 'limitless' logic in that, for example, our knowledge of health-related risks continues to grow, arguably making living healthily a much more fluid, 'always-on' enterprise than in the past. Fitness, meanwhile, increasingly borrows from health an emphasis on measuring the body against pre-established standards.

Each of these perspectives on fitness has merit. Recognizing that health and fitness are difficult to tease apart (as evidenced by the category of 'health and fitness' apps), the focus of this book lies with devices oriented towards capacities such as strength, flexibility, and cardiovascular endurance and/or towards a generally fit way of life through the incorporation of features like sleep tracking into one's daily routine. This is different from examining technologies focused mainly on established medical conditions, such as apps for insulin tracking among people with diabetes. Equally, the focus herein lies with the manner in which a fit lifestyle is characterized as a necessity, especially by those with fitness products to sell. This reflects Smith Maguire's emphasis on the cultural dimensions of fitness experience. As we shall see, the idea that fitness knows no bounds is relevant to this analysis as well. That one can always be fitter makes fitness a perfect ally for consumerism.

Theorizing technology

Theorizing technology is an even trickier proposition. There is value in the common understanding of technology as the application of science, but this perspective is ultimately much too narrow. Another way to address this matter is to consider theoretical traditions that are aimed, at least in part, at understanding technologies themselves and the significance of their production and use.

One such tradition we can label 'technology as repressive'. We have already heard from one of its more famous proponents. Neil Postman has seen something of a revitalization in recent times. *Amusing Ourselves to Death* was published in the mid-1980s, but its core message – that an American culture that had succumb to television's logic of sound bites and instantaneity could not sustain the type of thoughtful, detailed, and often protracted dialogue necessary for civil society to function properly – has earned newfound attention on the heels of Donald Trump's ascendancy to the American presidency (e.g., see Postman, 2017). Postman is interested mainly in technology as a means of communication. More to the point, he is concerned with technology's epistemological relevance, which is to say its bearing on the construction of truth. "In particular," Postman (1986) writes in *Amusing Ourselves to Death*, "I want to show that definitions of truth are derived, at least in part, from the character of the media of communication through which information is conveyed" (p. 17). *The form of communication necessarily affects its content*. The nuclear family on Postman's book cover was literally headless but metaphorically mindless: television's form makes content into meaningless junk, including content that should be informative and erudite. In all, technology is indeed a repressive force, one that has fomented our surrender, even death.

Another well-known contribution in this tradition is Herbert Marcuse's *One Dimensional Man* (1964), a text located squarely in the Marxist tradition. For Marx, alienation was a function of labour inequality. Through mass production, the proletariat is alienated from the fruits of its labour and from humankind's fundamental species-being. For Marcuse, the proliferation of false needs in consumer culture means that alienation is inescapable beyond the workplace as well. Writes Marcuse (1964),

> The productive apparatus and the goods and services which it produces 'sell' or impose the social system as a whole. The means of mass

transportation and communication, the commodities of lodging, food, and clothing, the irresistible output of the entertainment and information industry carry with them prescribed attitudes and habits, certain intellectual and emotional reactions which bind the consumers more or less pleasantly to the producers and, through the latter, to the whole.

(pp. 11–12)

What underpins this holistic form of social control is technological rationality – one might infer as much from the above passage. Technology is, more precisely, a mode of production for Marcuse (2009), as well as "the totality of instruments, devices, and contrivances which characterize the machine age" (p. 63). 'Technics' is the term Marcuse uses for the specific technical tools of industry, transportation, and communication. Marcuse's broad definition of technology reflects Jacques Ellul's (1964) use of the term 'technique' – something that includes machines but ultimately involves "the *totality of methods rationally arrived at and having absolute efficiency* (for a given stage of development) in *every* field of human activity" (p. xxv, emphasis in original). In both cases, the notion of technology as applied science is revealed to be inadequate in that social relations precede and inform technological development. Guy Debord likewise argues in *The Society of the Spectacle* (2014) that the spectacle is "a social relationship mediated by images" (p. 2). Again, in Debord's account, the language is rather grim. The technologically mediated spectacle amounts to the negation of life.

As a rejoinder to this first line of thinking, we can turn to that notable sceptic of repression hypotheses, Michel Foucault. At the core of Foucault's oeuvre sits his most famous line: "If power were never anything but repressive, if it never did anything but to say no, do you really think one would be brought to obey it?" He continues,

What makes power hold good, what makes it accepted, is simply the fact that it doesn't only weigh on us as a force that says no; it also traverses and produces things, it induces pleasure, forms of knowledge, produces discourse. It needs to be a productive network that runs through the whole social body, much more than a negative instance whose function is repression.

(Foucault, 2003, p. 307)

Foucault's work has the peculiar quality of being largely silent on modern technologies like television and, at the same time, using the term technology itself quite liberally. For Foucault, technology is not so much a thing-in-itself but rather a means of 'conducting conduct' – which is to say, a means for realizing what Foucault called 'governmentality'. For example, and as Steve Matthewman (2011) observes in making the case for Foucault as a theorist of technology, discipline in Foucault's work is a micropolitical technology aimed at the individual body. Biopower is a technology of security relevant to the population as a whole. In this formulation, something as broad as school-based PE is a governmental technology in that it aims to discipline the individual into shape in the interest of the nation state writ large (see Markula & Pringle, 2006). None of this should be taken to mean that Foucault entirely overlooked the role of specific (technological) instruments in the operation of power. In the history of medicine, for example, the stethoscope emboldened the medical gaze (Foucault, 2012; see Matthewman, 2011).

Nonetheless, the case for Foucault as a theorist of technology rests more on the legacy of his collective works than anything else. In a narrow sense, Foucault has become, along with Orwell, *the* theorist of surveillance studies in a time of proliferating information and communication technologies. More broadly, Foucault's legacy is seen in the work of those who have effectively sought to update his conception of governmentality, in part with technological change in mind. Gilles Deleuze's (1992) 'Postscript on the Societies of Control' accounts for the transition from the relatively enclosed, disciplinary spaces that preoccupied Foucault (prisons and medical clinics, for example) to more open forms of 'conducting conduct'. Different types of machines can be matched with different societies, Deleuze (1992) argues, though machines are not entirely deterministic of social arrangements. He continues,

> The old societies of sovereignty made use of simple machines – levers, pulleys, clocks; but the recent disciplinary societies equipped themselves with machines involving energy, with the passive danger of entropy and the active danger of sabotage; the societies of control operate with machines of a third type, computers, whose passive danger is jamming and whose active one is the introduction of viruses.
>
> (p. 6)

Said otherwise, whereas the factory was once a driver of and a perfect metaphor for capitalism – enclosed, productive, and localized – the factory has now given way to the flexible and dispersed *corporation*. The role of technology in control societies is variegated, but it includes helping once-confined institutions extend their reach. Chapter 4 herein shall make the case that the fitness gym, via fitness technologies, is one such institution.

Like Deleuze, and indeed drawing from Deleuze, Nikolas Rose (2007) has further developed Foucault's line of thinking as well, in his case in conceptualizing the contemporary politics of life itself. Foucault understands biopolitics as the combined means of sustaining the species body; it is "the taking charge of life" through, for example, the making of a new truth regime on sexuality (Foucault, 1990, p. 143). Rose accounts for the radical extension of such logic in the context of rapid technological development.

Contemporary biopolitics are not just a matter of establishing and promoting 'healthy' norms, but of guarding against susceptibility and enhancing virtually any imaginable capacity through technological intervention. 'Discipline and punish' gives way to 'screen and intervene' (Rose, 2008). "What is technology?" Rose (1996) asks. The response, again, takes us beyond technological instruments themselves:

> Technology, here, refers to any assembly structured by practical rationality governed by a more or less conscious goal . . . hybrid assemblages of knowledges, instruments, persons, systems of judgment, buildings and spaces, underpinned at the programmatic level by certain presuppositions and assumptions about human beings.
>
> (p. 26; cited in Rose, 2007, pp. 17–18; also see Brown & Webster, 2004)

Another line of thinking to consider under the 'technology as productive' mantle is the cultural studies tradition, especially its British iteration. A trademark of the Birmingham Centre for Contemporary Cultural Studies (CCCS) was the interest among CCCS scholars in eliciting lived accounts of consumer experience. The CCCS was different in this way from the Frankfurt School, of which Marcuse was a part. It makes sense that a more empirically oriented scholarly approach would not so easily equate consumerism with false consciousness.

When it comes to technology, Stuart Hall's (1993) 'Encoding, Decoding' essay is among the most important contributions in the cultural studies tradition. Hall conceived of communication as an integrated 'circuit of culture' composed of "linked but distinctive moments" (p. 91). It was, perhaps, unremarkable to say that media production involves material instruments and social relations, both brought together in the production of meaning. Yet 'Encoding, Decoding' is especially memorable for Hall's conception of how discourse is actively interpreted in *consumption*: "Before [a] message can have an 'effect' (however defined), satisfy a 'need' or be put to 'use', it must first be appropriated as a meaningful discourse and be meaningfully decoded" (p. 93). This formulation in turn inspired subsequent generations of research into audience experiences, especially in relation to TV programming, though other forms of communication were studied too (e.g., Ang, 1985; Gray, 1992; Lull, 1990; also see Alasuutari, 1999; Millington & Wilson, 2010). What emerges from this research is indeed a picture of constrained but still-active engagement with communication technology. The TV and the VCR, among other technologies, engendered various responses from consumers. As objects in themselves, they helped produce particular household relations as well (e.g., in affecting where families would physically gather).

The picture is complex enough, but there is a third tradition worth considering as well – Science and Technology Studies (STS). Bruno Latour's most succinct statement on technology is that technology is 'society made durable' (Latour, 1990). Yet this claim sits atop a nuanced critique of how social relations have long been conceived in scholarly accounts. The 'sociology of the social', as Latour (2005) calls it, assumes a pre-existing social structure (or some variant of this language) whose pre-existence helps us understand the subsequent existence of some specific social thing or process: the social explains the social. Latour's (preferred) 'sociology of associations' is based instead on a kind of epistemological flattening: the social is better understood as *socio-technical* in that it comprises interconnected chains of humans and non-humans. Technology is society made durable in that non-humans – a machine maybe – emerge out of the networked associations of other non-humans and people, and in turn help in holding society together. Indeed, and as shown in subsequent chapters, non-humans are constantly delegated the tasks and responsibilities once assigned to people themselves.

Among the many ways in which STS have proven influential is in helping to think through the literal articulations of people and things and what this means, in an ontological sense, for humankind. The posthumanism literature generally aims to de-centre humans in relation to various non-humans – machines included, but other parts of contemporary ecosystems as well (e.g., see Haraway, 2003). Tamar Sharon (2014) argues that Latour's concept of mediation, whereby non-humans hold the potential to actively alter meaning and experience, helps pave a pathway between dystopic and liberal accounts of posthumanism. The dystopic view sees technology as something that impinges on human activity from 'the outside'. The liberal perspective focuses on human uses of technology aimed at mastering 'outside' environments. Both accounts are flawed, Sharon (2014) argues, in regarding people and things as fundamentally discrete. She advocates a view instead whereby "the human is seen as originally existing in relation to and as dependent on its technologies, which it always already incorporates" (p. 81). Technology is born from the 'folding together' (Latour, 1999) of humans and non-humans and subsequently helps engender further articulations of this kind.

Taken together, these three traditions of technology criticism are in many ways at odds. Acknowledging that the 'repressive' vs. 'productive' binary is somewhat artificial – for example, those working within the Foucauldian tradition are quite clearly concerned with the inequalities that arise or are solidified through technology-enabled forms of surveillance – there is nonetheless a difference between construing technology as central to either the negation or the optimization of life. Likewise, while the Science and Technology Studies tradition might be understood in one sense as a 'middle ground' between the repressive and productive traditions, STS has been critiqued, and Latour's contributions especially have been critiqued, for disregarding the power dynamics of lived experience that are so central to the repressive and productive points of view (see Matthewman, 2011). Said otherwise, for

Marcuse, modern life is alienating; for Foucault, modern power is everywhere and productive; for Latour (1993), we have never been modern to begin with, entangled as we are with non-humans of various kinds.

At the very least, what can be drawn from these traditions is that technology is not simply applied science. Technology involves tangible 'things' in their own right, but it equally involves the many 'things' and relationships that inform technological development in the first place and emerge out of the actual uses of technologies in the end. Technology, like fitness, is a process and an outcome. In the spirit of Latour's body of work, the goal of subsequent chapters is, in part, to account for the many 'actants' that suddenly appear when we scrutinize otherwise 'blackboxed' technologies. But this assembling of actants shall also be construed as *productive*; it has a purpose. More than that: it is productive in a way that aligns with already-existing discourses. This book is inspired by the STS view that the important role of non-humans in making society durable has been largely underestimated and underrepresented in scholarly accounts. But it rejects the idea that accounting for context is necessarily tautological – a case of the social explaining the social – and thus problematic (also see Millington & Wilson, 2016). To paraphrase Marx, people and technologies make their own histories, but not under conditions of their own choosing. Thomas Lemke (2015) makes the argument that the STS and governmentality traditions are not so opposed. The 'conduct of conduct' involves governance *through* both humans and non-humans with the aim of governing both humans and non-humans in turn. The specific case made herein is that fitness technologies, as productive assemblages, must be understood as products of our present-day (and already-existing) neoliberal conjuncture in particular; in turn, they fortify neoliberalism's very existence. As Lemke (2001) says elsewhere, neoliberalism, in imposing a market logic on life as a whole, is, above all, "a political project that endeavours to create a social reality that it suggests already exists" (p. 203). Self-tracking both reflects and creates a vision of entrepreneurial subjectivity.

And yet, as outlined in the Conclusion Chapter of this book especially, this conception of fitness technologies does not mean we should leave the repression tradition behind entirely. Postman's sceptical outlook on the state of technology will be revisited in assessing the problems that arise as we are urged with increasing frequency to amuse ourselves to life.

Fitness, technology and society

There are many ways to understand fitness and technology. Certainly, there are many ways to study them too. Let us begin by considering what *Amusing Ourselves to Life* does *not* aim to do.

This book does not attempt to assess the validity of Fitbit products, Wii Fit, and other technologies of this kind – validity in the sense of their accuracy in measuring the body and one's daily activities. Work of this kind would require a positivist paradigmatic view. Indeed, such work exists and is important in understanding the new fitness boom in its full scope. Studies to date have come to mixed conclusions on the accuracy of interactive health and fitness devices. As said recently in *The New York Times*, when it comes to the accuracy of fitness trackers, the jury is still out (McPhate, 2016).

What *is* clear is that commercial fitness technologies are not perfect. For example, Case et al. (2015) examined a rather basic function – step counting – in ten technologies, including hardware made by Fitbit and software apps running on Apple and Samsung devices. Results were compared against direct (i.e., human) observation of steps taken: "the relative difference in mean step count ranged from –0.3% to 1.0% for the pedometer and accelerometers, –22.7 % to –1.5% for the wearable devices, and –6.7% to 6.2% for smartphone applications" (p. 625). These results were generally consistent with 500-step and 1500-step trials. The –22.7% result should perhaps come with an exclamation point at the end, as this is quite a large under-estimation of steps taken. But, in all, the authors conclude that "many smartphone applications and wearable devices were accurate for tracking step counts" (p. 625). *Not perfect, but generally fair.* Jung-Min Lee, Youngwon Kim, and Gregory Welk (2014) went further in assessing four physical activity types – sedentary, walking, running, and moderate-to-vigorous activities (e.g., playing basketball) – in 30 healthy men and 30 healthy women. Eight wearable products were tested, again including those from prominent sellers such as Fitbit and Nike. With the exception of one device (the Basis B1 Band), measures of energy expenditure were deemed 'reasonable' on the whole – which is to say within approximately 10%–15% error when compared to a non-commercial, lab-grade technology (also see Diaz et al., 2015; Nelson et al., 2016; Takacs et al., 2014).

Meanwhile, in a study of exergaming among adolescents and younger and older adults, Graves et al. (2010) found that energy expenditure and heart rate were significantly greater during Wii Fit activities (yoga, muscle conditioning, balance, and aerobics) than in handheld (i.e., sedentary) gaming, but that these same measures were significantly *lower* than those for treadmill walking and jogging. In other words, if the question is whether exergames are good for you or not, one's point of comparison is important. That said, enjoyment in exergaming is another matter to consider. Enjoyment in Wii Fit activities was comparable to, if not greater than, what it was for handheld gaming and treadmill exercise. The 'gaming' side of exergaming might thus be a draw to those looking to get fit.

Research of this kind is undoubtedly worth pursuing. And while the objectivity of such research should not be taken for granted – for instance, the verdict on what is reasonable in terms of margin for error is debatable – the main reason that research into the *significance* of the new fitness boom is needed is that accuracy is not the sole criterion for success with health and fitness technologies. In the fictional scenario that 100% accuracy was achieved, would it mean activity tracking is unquestionably a social 'good'? The answer is quite clearly 'no' if we consider evidence showing that self-tracking can trade intrinsic motivation for extrinsic motivation, thus making exercise feel more like work (Etkin, 2016).

It need be said too that the chapters that follow this introductory chapter do not examine fitness cultures and experiences in their totality. Fitness is a constantly evolving field – as seen recently, for example, in the rise to prominence of CrossFit, a fitness regimen involving functional movements performed at high intensity (e.g., see Heywood, 2015). There have been several social scientific assessments of fitness and its implications in recent years (e.g., see Andreasson & Johansson, 2014; Pronger, 2002; Sassatelli, 2010). *Amusing Ourselves to Life* must be understood alongside these other texts to gain a bigger picture sense of what fitness means at this moment in time and what it has meant historically as well. It is worth noting too that this analysis draws from English-language resources exclusively and as such paints a picture of fitness in the Global North, and especially in Canada, the United States, and the United Kingdom.

Finally, and in a third sense, this book is by no means the final word even on health and fitness technologies themselves. A theme of Chapter 2 is that the technology sector's need for perpetual innovation has now been brought to bear on the pursuit of fit living. What this means for this book is that fitness technologies in general are sure to have evolved further by the time this analysis is read. Even products considered in specific terms in subsequent chapters are likely to have taken on new functionalities and discarded older ones. This is just one contribution in the ongoing study of fitness technology.

What this book *is* is an attempt to critically examine Fitness 2.0 – critical in the sense not simply of identifying what is wrong with health and fitness technologies, but in the sense of considering what we know of the logics and materials through which they are built, the ways in which they are represented to the public (which is to say, their potential consumers), their regulation by governments, their use by individual consumers or in institutional contexts, and, above all, the implications of all of this for what health and fitness mean at the current moment in time. In many ways, this is a *sympathetic* reading of fitness technologies, mainly in that this book largely takes technology merchants at their word. Recognizing that the jury is still out on devices like Fitbit activity trackers, the chapters that follow generally assume that technologies of this kind do what they are said to do in promotional materials. To assume that the Fitbit Surge tracks, 'datafies', and represents activity and the body as proclaimed in Fitbit marketing (and as said earlier) allows consideration of how fitness technologies have changed over time and how fit living is, at the current moment, said to be achievable.

The chapters that follow draw from a range of sources in carrying out this critical examination. Most of all, they draw from the growing body of social scientific literature devoted to the interactive and personalized devices that are changing the fitness landscape in rather profound ways. This is supplemented with information and examples drawn from marketing materials (promotional websites in particular), press releases announcing new product releases or corporate relations in the fitness/technology industries, historical texts outlining what fitness has meant in past eras, and news media reporting on trends in health and fitness – with 'news media' understood broadly so as to include niche technology sites (e.g., TechCrunch) and more mainstream news organizations (e.g., the Wall Street Journal). Sourcing includes references to when online materials were accessed with the understanding that technologies (and their descriptions) are indeed always evolving.

The remainder of this book unfolds through six overlapping chapters.

The purpose of **Chapter 1** is to historicize the new fitness boom. The analysis at this time specifically considers how health and fitness were understood at three key historical 'moments': ancient Greece, which gave us both the gymnasium and the idea that physical activity could be directed towards bodily ideals; the physical culture movement of the late 1800s and early 1900s, at which time the moral dimensions of fit living were reinscribed; and finally the first fitness boom of the 1970s and 1980s, a time when fitness became a commercial pursuit more so than ever and fitness was understood through a moral lens yet again. Thinking across these different moments in time, Chapter 1 ultimately presents a story of technological change. Whereas ancient Greeks relied on simple tools to get fit and physical culturalists sold the merits of simple machines, the first fitness boom brought electronic fitness technologies to the fore, paving the way for today's interactive, digital devices.

Chapter 2 turns to the political economy of fitness technologies with the aim of unearthing the various 'actants' behind the arrival of the new fitness boom. This chapter begins with a case study of Nintendo's incorporation of health and fitness motifs into its product catalogue in the mid-2000s with the release of the aforementioned Wii console. The Nintendo narrative is compelling in its own right, given that it signals how technologies that have long been demonized for their health and fitness implications are now being built with healthy outcomes in mind. The broader aim of Chapter 2, however, is to draw lessons from Nintendo's story, including the lesson that the fitness and technology sectors have now effectively merged together, forming a fitness-technology complex.

Having examined the political economic side of the fitness-technology landscape, **Chapter 3** and **Chapter 4** assess the functionalities of fitness technologies such as wearable activity trackers. Chapter 3 deals mainly with how surveillance manifests in the new fitness boom. Drawing on

Haggerty and Ericson's (2000) concept of the surveillant assemblage, the analysis at this time considers how different surveillance modalities are now brought together in the quest for technology-enabled optimization. Chapter 4 continues this analysis but focuses specifically on mobility as it pertains to the new fitness boom. This is the 'always-on' dimension of fitness experience referred to earlier; surveillance arises not only in many forms but also anywhere and anytime. Chapter 4 is also where matters such as privacy and data security are addressed in this book in greatest detail. Consideration is also given to the nature of regulation in the new fitness boom.

Chapter 5 deals with what is known at present about consumer experiences in the time of Fitness 2.0. This chapter again begins with a Nintendo case study, though in this instance it considers lessons learned from a study of exergaming in Canadian retirement centres. From there, Chapter 5 deals with what is known about self-tracking (e.g., through mobile, wearable technologies) and about fitness dialogue on social media such as Twitter. The chapter concludes with a discussion as to how the common conclusion that consumers are inherently active and creative in their uses of fitness technologies sits alongside the problematizing of empowerment discourses that pervade the critical literature on the concept of healthism.

Finally, in reflecting on the analyses presented throughout this book, the **Conclusion Chapter** outlines eight characteristics of the new fitness boom – the aim being to both assess contemporary fitness technologies and to identify trends that can help in foreseeing where fitness is headed in years to come. The significance of fitness technologies is also assessed at this time with help from the theoretical traditions outlined earlier. Rather than a fitness revolution, fitness technologies are deemed instruments of governmentality: this is the conduct of conduct re-conceptualized in and for neoliberal times. That said, while fitness technologies are seen as productive in this regard, the other theoretical traditions referred to earlier are revisited in this concluding chapter as well. That we can now amuse ourselves to life is looked upon sceptically in the spirit of Postman's *Amusing Ourselves to Death*.

References

Alasuutari, P. (1999). Introduction: Three phases in reception studies. In P. Alasuutari (Ed.), *Rethinking the media audience: The new agenda* (pp. 1–21). Thousand Oaks: Sage.

Andreasson, J. & Johansson, T. (2014). *The global gym: Gender, health and pedagogies*. New York: Palgrave Macmillan.

Ang, I. (1985). *Watching Dallas: Soap opera and melodramatic imagination*. London: Methuen.

Bauman, Z. (1995). *Life in fragments: Essays in postmodern morality*. Oxford: Blackwell Publishers.

Bauman, Z. (2011). *Liquid life*. Cambridge: Polity Press.

Brown, N. & Webster, A. (2004). *New medical technologies and society: Reordering life*. Cambridge: Polity.

BusinessWire. (2017). Fitbit adds software tools that deliver inspiration, personalization and smarter guidance. Retrieved 19 February 2017 from www.businesswire.com/news/home/20170105005233/en/Fitbit-Adds-Software-Tools-Deliver-Inspiration-Personalization.

Case, M.A., Burwick, H.A., Volpp, K.G. & Patel, M.S. (2015). Accuracy of smartphone applications and wearable devices for tracking physical activity data. *JAMA*, *313*(6), 625–626.

Citrix. (2015). Mobile analytics report. Retrieved from www.citrix.com/blogs/2015/02/10/key-takeaways-for-enterprises-from-the-2015-citrix-mobile-analytics-report/.

Debord, G. (2014). *Society of the spectacle*. Berkeley: Bureau of Public Secrets.

Deleuze, G. (1992). Postscript on the societies of control. *October*, *59*, 3–7.

Diaz, K.M., Krupka, D.J., Chang, M.J., Peacock, J., Ma, Y., Goldsmith, J., Schwartz, J.E. & Davidson, K.W. (2015). Fitbit®: An accurate and reliable device for wireless physical activity tracking. *International Journal of Cardiology*, *185*, 138–140.

The Economist. (2016). Things are looking app: Mobile health apps are becoming more capable and potentially rather useful. Retrieved 19 February 2017 from www.economist.com/news/business/21694523-mobile-health-apps-are-becoming-more-capable-and-potentially-rather-useful-things-are-looking.

Eisenman, P.A. & Barnett, C.R. (1979). Physical fitness in the 1950s and 1970s: Why did one fail and the other boom? *Quest*, *31*(1), 114–122.

Ellul, J. (1964). *The technological society*. New York: Vintage Books.

Etkin, J. (2016). The hidden cost of personal quantification. *Journal of Consumer Research*, *42*(6), 967–984.

Fitbit Inc. (2017). Surge. Retrieved 19 February 2017 from www.fitbit.com/uk/surge.

Foucault, M. (1990). *The history of sexuality, Volume 1: An introduction*. London: Penguin.

Foucault, M. (2003). Truth and power. In P. Rabinow & N.S. Rose (Eds.), *The essential Foucault: Selections from essential works of Foucault, 1954–1984* (pp. 300–318). New York: New Press.

Foucault, M. (2012). *The birth of the clinic*. New York: Routledge.

Gard, M. (2011). Truth, belief and the cultural politics of obesity scholarship and public health policy. *Critical Public Health*, *21*(1), 37–48.

Glanze, W.D. (1986). *Mosby's medical and nursing dictionary*. St. Louis: Mosby.

Graves, L.E., Ridgers, N.D., Williams, K., Stratton, G., Atkinson, G. & Cable, N.T. (2010). The physiological cost and enjoyment of Wii Fit in adolescents, young adults, and older adults. *Journal of Physical Activity and Health*, *7*(3), 393–401.

Gray, A. (1992). *Video playtime: The gendering of a leisure technology*. New York: Routledge.

Haggerty, K.D. & Ericson, R.V. (2000). The surveillant assemblage. *British Journal of Sociology*, *51*(4), 605–622.

Hall, S. (1993). Encoding, decoding. In S. During (Ed.), *The cultural studies reader* (pp. 90–103). London: Routledge.

Haraway, D.J. (2003). *The companion species manifesto: Dogs, people, and significant otherness*. Chicago: Prickly Paradigm Press.

Heywood, L. (2015). The CrossFit sensorium: Visuality, affect and immersive sport. *Paragraph*, *38*(1), 20–36.

HM Government. (2015). Sporting future: A new strategy for an active nation. Retrieved 23 June 2017 from https://www.gov.uk/government/publications/sporting-future-a-new-strategy-for-an-active-nation.

Jones, S.E. & Thiruvathukal, G.K. (2012). *Codename revolution: The Nintendo Wii platform.* Cambridge: MIT Press.

Lake, A.A., Townshend, T.G. & Alvanides, S. (Eds.). (2010). *Obesogenic environments: Complexities, perceptions and objective measures.* Chichester: Wiley-Blackwell.

Lamkin, P. (2016). Wearable tech market to be worth $34 billion by 2020. Retrieved 19 February 2017 from www.forbes.com/sites/paullamkin/2016/02/17/wearable-tech-market-to-be-worth-34-billion-by-2020/#2265c48e3fe3.

Latham, A. (2015). The history of a habit: Jogging as a palliative to sedentariness in 1960s America. *Cultural Geographies, 22*(1), 103–126.

Latour, B. (1990). Technology is society made durable. *The Sociological Review, 38*(S1), 103–131.

Latour, B. (1993). *We have never been modern.* Cambridge: Harvard Press.

Latour, B. (1999). *Pandora's hope: Essays on the reality of science studies.* Cambridge: Harvard Press.

Latour, B. (2005). *Reassembling the social: An introduction to actor-network-theory.* Oxford: Oxford Press.

Lay, K. (2015). Obesity as dangerous as terror threat, warns medical chief. Retrieved 19 February 2017 from www.thetimes.co.uk/tto/health/news/article4638602.ece.

Lee, J.-M., Kim, Y. & Welk, G.J. (2014). Validity of consumer-based physical activity monitors. *Medicine & Science in Sports & Exercise, 46*(9), 1840–1848.

Lemke, T. (2001). 'The birth of bio-politics': Michel Foucault's lecture at the Collège _de France on neo-liberal governmentality. *Economy and Society, 30*(2), 190–207.

Lemke, T. (2015). New materialisms: Foucault and the 'government of things'. *Theory, Culture & Society, 32*(4), 3–25.

Lorinc, J., Tossell, I. & el Akkad, O. (2010). The age of the app. Retrieved 19 May 2016 from www.theglobeandmail.com/report-on-business/rob-magazine/the-age-of-the-app/article1510836/?cid=art-rail-economy.

Lull, J. (1990). *Inside family viewing: Ethnographic research on television's audience.* New York: Routledge.

Lupton, D. (2012). *Fat.* New York: Routledge.

Marcuse, H. (1964). *One dimensional man: Studies in the ideology of advanced industrial society.* London: Routledge & Kegan Paul Limited.

Marcuse, H. (2009). Social implications of technology. In D.M. Kaplan (Ed.), *Readings in the philosophy of technology* (pp. 63–79). Lanham: Rowman & Littlefield Publishers, Inc.

Markula, P. & Pringle, R. (2006). *Foucault, sport & exercise: Power, knowledge and transforming the self.* New York: Routledge.

Matthewman, S. (2011). *Technology and social theory.* New York: Palgrave Macmillan.

Maud, P.J. (2006). Fitness assessment defined. In P.J. Maud & C. Foster (Eds.), *Physiological assessment of human fitness* (Second edition, pp. 1–8). Champaign: Human Kinetics.

McPhate, M. (2016). Just how accurate are Fitbits? The jury is out. Retrieved 17 February 2017 from www.nytimes.com/2016/05/26/technology/personaltech/fitbit-accuracy.html?_r=1.

Millington, B. & Wilson, B. (2010). Media consumption and the contexts of physical culture: Methodological reflections on a 'third generation' study of media audiences. *Sociology of Sport Journal*, 27(1), 30–53.

Millington, B. & Wilson, B. (2016 [Online First]). Contested terrain and terrain that contests: Donald Trump, golf's environmental politics, and a challenge to anthropocentrism in Physical Cultural Studies. *International Review for the Sociology of Sport*. DOI: https://doi.org/10.1177/1012690216631541.

Mitroff, S. (2015). Under Armour scoops up health apps MyFitnessPal and Endomondo. Retrieved 19 February 2017 from www.cnet.com/uk/news/under-armour-scoops-up-health-apps-myfitnesspal-and-endomondo/.

Nelson, M.B., Kaminsky, L.A., Dickin, D.C. & Montoye, A.H. (2016). Validity of consumer-based physical activity monitors for specific activity types. *Medicine and Science in Sports and Exercise*, 48(8), 1619–1628.

Nintendo. (2016). Top selling software units. Retrieved 15 February 2017 from www. nintendo.co.jp/ir/en/sales/software/wii.html.

ParticipACTION. (2016). Are Canadian Kids too tired to move? Results from the 2016 report card. Retrieved 16 February 2017 from www.participaction. com/sites/default/files/downloads/2016%20ParticipACTION%20Report%20 Card%20-%20Presentation.pdf.

Pierce, D. (2016). How Under Armour plans to turn your clothes into gadgets. Retrieved 19 May 2016 from www.wired.com/2016/01/under-armour-healthbox/.

Postman, A. (2017). My dad predicted Trump in 1985 – It's not Orwell, he warned, it's Brave New World. Retrieved 18 February 2017 from www.theguardian.com/ media/2017/feb/02/amusing-ourselves-to-death-neil-postman-trump-orwell-huxley.

Postman, N. (1986). *Amusing ourselves to death: Public discourse in the age of show business*. New York: Penguin Books.

Pronger, B. (2002). *Body fascism: Salvation in the technology of physical fitness*. Toronto: University of Toronto Press.

Radar, B. (1991). The quest for self-sufficiency and the new strenuosity: Reflections on the strenuous life of the 1970s and the 1980s. *Journal of Sport History*, 18(2), 255–266.

Rose, N. (1996). *Inventing our selves: Psychology, power, and personhood*. New York: Cambridge University Press.

Rose, N. (2007). *The politics of life itself: Biomedicine, power, and subjectivity in the twenty-first century*. Princeton: Princeton University Press.

Rose, N. (2008). Race, risk and medicine in the age of 'your own personal genome'. *BioSocieties*, 3(4), 423–439.

Sassatelli, R. (2010). *Fitness culture: Gyms and the commercialisation of discipline and fun*. New York: Palgrave Macmillan.

Scheerder, J., Breedveld, K. & Borgers, J. (2015). Who is doing a run with the running boom? The growth and governance of one of Europe's most popular sport activities. In J. Scheerder, K. Breedveld & J. Borgers (Eds.), *Running across Europe: The rise and size of one of the largest sport markets* (pp. 1–27). New York: Palgrave Macmillan.

Sharon, T. (2014). *Human nature in an age of biotechnology: The case for mediated posthumanism*. New York: Springer.

Smith Maguire, J. (2008). *Fit for consumption: Sociology and the business of fitness*. New York: Routledge.

Standing Senate Committee on Social Affairs, Science and Technology. (2016). Obesity in Canada: A whole-of-society approach for a healthier Canada. Retrieved

19 February 2017 from https://sencanada.ca/content/sen/committee/421/SOCI/Reports/2016-02-25_Revised_report_Obesity_in_Canada_e.pdf.

Takacs, J., Pollock, C.L., Guenther, J.R., Bahar, M., Napier, C. & Hunt, M.A. (2014). Validation of the Fitbit One activity monitor device during treadmill walking. *Journal of Science and Medicine in Sport*, 17(5), 496–500.

Terry, K. (2015). Number of health apps soars, but use does not always follow. Retrieved 17 February 2017 from www.medscape.com/viewarticle/851226.

Toon, E. & Golden, J. (2002). 'Live clean, think clean, and don't go to burlesque shows': Charles Atlas as health advisor. *Journal of the History of Medicine*, 57, 39–60.

Tremblay, M.S. & Lloyd, M. (2010). Physical literacy measurement: The missing piece. *Physical and Health Education Journal*, 76(1), 26–30.

Turkle, S. (2008). Always-on/always-on-you: The tethered self. In J.E. Katz (Ed.), *Handbook of mobile communication studies* (pp. 121–137). Cambridge: MIT Press.

U.S. Department of Health & Human Services. (n.d.a). President's council on fitness, sports & nutrition. Retrieved 17 February 2017 from www.fitness.gov/about-pcf sn/our-history/.

U.S. Department of Health & Human Services. (n.d.b). Surgeon general's healthy apps challenge: About the winners. Retrieved 19 February 2017 from www.surgeongeneral.gov/news/2012/02/sg_healthy_app_challenge-winners.html.

World Health Organization. (2017). Constitution of WHO: Principles. Retrieved 17 February 2017 from www.who.int/about/mission/en/.

Chapter 1

Historicizing fitness technology

> Who would have thought not long ago that Oscar Wilde, the apostle of dainty estheticism, the wit and poet, fêted everywhere and even worshipped at times by people of position and discernment – who would have dreamed it even? – would come to sweating on a prison treadmill?

So began the article 'Oscar Wilde on a Treadmill', published on 23 June 1895 in the American newspaper *The Chicago Sunday Tribune* (1895, p. 42). Wilde, the famous Irish poet, playwright, and writer, had been sentenced in England in the same year to two years' hard labour, the maximum allowable penalty, for the crime of indecency – in this case a synonym for homosexuality. Wilde suffered terribly in prison. As Vybarr Cregan Reid (2012) recounts, Victorian-era sentences of 'hard labour' in prison could be traced back to the 1778 Hard Labour Bill and the recommendation therein to build 'Hard Labour Houses' for punishing and humiliating prisoners. In the 1800s, the treadmill, or treadwheel as it was sometimes called, was devised and implemented in prisons as a way of achieving these ends. The treadmill, continued the *Tribune*'s (1895) review of Wilde's plight, was the bugaboo of the English prisoner:

> It is almost barbaric in its severity and savors somewhat of the torture inflicted upon unfortunates 500 years ago. It is shaped somewhat like the wheel of a stern-wheel steamer or the paddle-wheel of a ferry-boat, except that the treadmill is considerably wider than they are. . . . When all is ready the prisoner jumps upon one of the steps of the wheel and grasps the bar with his hands. . . . The weight of the men turns the wheel, and as they sink down on one foot they must step up to the next float when it comes round. It is much like climbing a particularly nasty flight of steep stairs with no ending at the top.
>
> (p. 42)

Though befallen by life-threatening exhaustion, Wilde survived his sentence of Sisyphean labour. He died, however, at age 46, just three years after his release from prison. That the treadmill, a device that perhaps hastened Wilde's demise, is now used in households and fitness gyms the world over for *improving* health is an irony not lost on Reid (2012).

* * * * *

This chapter examines historical logics, practices, and technologies that underpin contemporary fitness practices. It focuses in particular on the nature and significance of fitness technologies at three historical 'moments': ancient Greece; the physical culture movement of the late 1800s and early 1900s; and the (first) fitness boom of the 1970s and 1980s. This is undoubtedly a selective history of fitness and fitness technologies. It would be impossible in this space to deliver an exhaustive account along these lines. The point instead is to demonstrate that present-day fitness technologies have a protracted – indeed, ancient – history and that the technologies of earlier eras in many ways presaged the new fitness boom dealt with in subsequent chapters. The term fitness is used throughout this chapter to signify activities related to strength, endurance, flexibility and the like, recognizing that other terms have been used over time (e.g., training) for a similar purpose.

In historicizing the present, this chapter plots a path of technological development: from *basic tools* like the pre-modern dumbbells of ancient Greece to *mechanical machines* like the door-attachable resistance apparatuses of the physical culture movement to *electronic technologies* like the cycling and rowing simulators of the late-twentieth-century fitness boom. To be sure, these technologies are not tied exclusively to particular moments in time – dumbbells still exist alongside treadmills, for example. The aim of this chapter is to outline how certain technologies gained cachet at given historical moments against the backdrop of wider contextual factors. For example, the technologies used to sculpt muscular bodies at the turn of the twentieth century need be understood as part of a context where musculature was believed to be in peril as a result of industrialization.

The chapter proceeds through four subsequent sections. The first three of these deal, respectively, with the historical moments referenced earlier. The final section assesses points of continuity and disruption across these moments, the most notable of which is the lasting idea that pursuing a fit body and a fit way of life is a *moral* responsibility. The final section of the chapter also revisits the case of Oscar Wilde and the exercise treadmill – that foe of the English convict turned friend of the fitness enthusiast.

The ancient gym

The through-line from past to present fitness practices is often traced to Classical Era Greece, given, as Roy Shephard (2015) writes, that the ancient Greeks famously created the Olympic Games and were concerned more generally with systematizing and institutionalizing health practices, including physical activity. Indeed, documentary evidence for the first gymnasia dates from the sixth century BCE. The Akademia (Academy), founded by Peisistratos (d. *c.* 527 BCE), son of Hippocrates, and open to freeborn male Athenians, was Greece's first 'public' gymnasium (Chaline, 2015).

The Greek word *gymnazein* means 'to exercise naked' – something that surely vindicates many of the outfits worn by today's fitness enthusiasts. But this should not be taken to mean that the earliest of gyms were technology-free spaces. The body was not bare. In one sense, the *kynodesme* was a key part of the male athlete's kit. Effectively an ancient jockstrap, the *kynodesme* was a leather thong that kept the penis stable during exercise. In another sense, the body was treated in a way that reflected scientific knowledge of the day. Oil and dust were applied for physiological purposes before physical activity began, the idea being that substances of this kind could help guard against excessive sweat, thus keeping one's bodily fluids in balance: "Clay disinfected and prevented excessive sweat; terracotta opened the pores, thereby promoting perspiration; and asphalt was heating" (Chaline, 2015, pp. 25–26).

In another sense still, the ancient Greeks are usually given credit for pioneering modern weight training equipment (Todd, 2003), even if the assistive implement famously employed by the Greek strongman Milo de Crotona – lifting a bull on one's shoulders, something Milo is alleged to have achieved by carrying the animal daily from the time it was young – has not stood the test of time. As Jan Todd (2003) recounts, by the fifth century BCE, the Greeks were using three main weight implements in training: "The diskos and javelin were thrown for distance, while the handheld *alteres* or *halteres* were used as a jumping aide and for muscle building" (p. 66). Halteres are perhaps the most compelling of these technologies in the sense that they stand as forerunners to modern-day dumbbells. Invented by pentathletes, halteres were generally made of stone, lead, or metal, and usually weighed between 3.5 to 5.5 pounds. Their purpose in jumping was to guide the hands, the logic being that this in turn would help keep the feet in good form (Sweet, 1987). Waldo Sweet (1987) adds that large halteres were used to exercise the arms and shoulders and that round ones were put to use in strengthening the fingers (also see Roach, 2008). Todd (2003) further remarks on the staying power of halteres in noting that there is evidence to suggest that the Romans copied the Greeks in using technologies of this kind in training.

Thus, in many ways, the ancient Greeks were fitness-technology pioneers, particularly in their use of simple tools for the purpose of training. But what is important in hindsight is not just the innovativeness associated with ancient Greek culture but also the contextualized nature of exercise technologies. It makes sense that halteres, among other devices, were used for gaining an edge in competition given the tremendous material rewards at stake in events such as the Olympic Games. Writes Chaline (2015), "Victory in competition brought the athlete an exalted position in his native city, one that elevated him well beyond the status of his fellow citizens and associated him with the gods themselves" (p. 32; also see Hubbard, 2008). Fitness was entwined with celebrity culture – something that, as we shall see, fitness luminaries in later centuries would quite literally capitalize upon.

As suggested earlier, fitness was also contextualized in the sense that bodywork was part of a broader project aimed at understanding life in scientific terms. As mythology increasingly ceded ground to evidence-based medicine, purposeful exercise was valued as a form of therapy. Hippocrates, for example, saw disease as a product of lifestyle and environment, as opposed to ancestral curses or divine punishment. This, in turn, paved the way towards advocating participation in activities such as wrestling while clothed in dust to avoid overheating (Kritikos et al., 2009; cited in Shephard, 2015, p. 192). At the same time, and by Shephard's (2015) account, for ancient Greeks, "Perfection of the body was seen as important to development of the mind" (p. 195). For Plato, optimizing health meant balancing mind and body. Plato went so far as to establish his school at the Academy, thus tying intellectual pursuits with the term 'academy' forever more.

Yet perhaps the most compelling point in contextualizing ancient fitness practices involves the Greek gymnasium's status as a site for sculpting a (male) body of 'ideal' proportions. Sculptures memorializing Greek athletes show well-defined muscles, "exemplifying in monumental form an ideal male body to which all aspired" (Lee, 2015, p. 59). As detailed by Mireille Lee (2015), exercise practices were in fact linked to a wider regimen of healthy behaviours called *diaita*, inclusive of diet and hygiene as well. When it came to diet, both over- and under-indulgence in eating were derided; obesity, for example, was satirized in comedy. Taken together, and remembering that women were barred from gymnasia, and thus the exercise and bathing sites therein, the ideal body stemming from adherence to a daily lifestyle regimen was male, muscular, and tanned; "its opposite was the female body, fleshy and pale" (Lee, 2015, p. 62). Importantly, and in a theme that shall run throughout this chapter and book in general, bodywork was furthermore tied to *moral* virtue – "a fine body could not be sorted with anything but a fine soul" (Chaline, 2015, p. 35).

Don't be a criminal: fitness as physical culture

Thus, in ancient Greece, technologies were brought together with emerging scientific knowledge and with broader exercise, dietary, and hygienic regimens in the pursuit of 'virtuous' ways of living. Bodywork certainly did not disappear with the fall of the Greek and Roman Empires. As Shephard (2015) writes, for example, during the Renaissance, ancient Greek ideals glorifying the body were taken up anew by scientists, artists, and poets. Physical education at this time became a place for bodily exertion with the aim of inuring (male) students to the physical hardships that awaited in battle. Even so, in tracing a through-line from present to past, the turn of the twentieth century stands out as yet another important moment in the history of fitness technologies. As Oscar Wilde climbed his infinite staircase, a wider physical culture movement was afoot.

As the name 'physical culture' intimates, the physical culture movement was in one sense about promoting different forms of physical activity – gymnastics, calisthenics, weight training, and competitive sports among them (Churchill, 2008). Yet physical culturalists were apt as well to think broadly when it came to fit living. For example, in his 1897 text, *Sandow on Physical Training*, the Prussian-born strongman Eugen Sandow weaved together his own mythology – a drawing on p. 98 of his book shows a man, presumably Sandow, balancing himself on two chairs, *and balancing a horse and adult rider on a board across his mid-section* – with didactic instruction on exercise, diet, and hygiene, among other matters. Sandow's contemporary, Bernarr Macfadden, was equally ostentatious, and equally keen on promoting constant attention to the quest for self-betterment (e.g., see Macfadden, 1915).

In terms of technology, the physical culture movement is significant in that it witnessed a shift from simple tools like halteres to *simple machines* – which is to say, mechanical devices designed mainly for resistance training through features like cables and pulleys. This is not to say that the hand-held tools of times' past were suddenly irrelevant. The Milo Adjustable Barbell, for example, was available for those looking to 'shape up'. Echoing the mythologized exercise regimen of Milo de Crotona, though replacing a growing animal with an adjustable barbell, the Milo Barbell was 'scientific' and 'progressive' in nature and was allegedly tried and tested by strongmen of the day (Green, 1986). Implements like gymnastics wands (for bending and stretching exercises) and Indian clubs (literally adopted from India via British imperialism, and used in ways similar to gymnastic wands) were likewise popular at the time (Todd, 2003).

But mechanical devices grew more prominent as well, in part through the commercial efforts of celebrity physical culture icons. The strongman Eugen Sandow was at the forefront of this trend, as his body was allegedly made possible by his use of intricate fitness apparatuses. The 1894 text, *Sandow on Physical Training: A Study in the Perfect Type of the Human Form*, was penned under Sandow's direction and supervision and named with characteristic modesty. Therein, author G. Mercer Adam (1894) describes a 'leg machine' used by Sandow alongside dumbbells and barbells in training:

> The machine consists of a base-board or platform, from five to six feet in length, having at either end an upright post or standard, secured by screws to the baseboard, and capped by ferrules with attached hooks or eyes, and a cross-bar for the hands to rest upon and give steadiness to the upright posts. About the middle of the cross-bar or brace, and a little apart, are two fixed hooks upon which are hung stirrups, connected by one or more rubber straps or elastic cables; into these stirrups the feet

are placed for the purpose of exercise, either by a direct up-and-down tread or by alternate lateral thrusts to the outer base of the machine.

(p. 236)

Adam's description of the leg machine is instructive first in showing the *constituent* technologies brought together with the body in the quest to strengthen the legs: upright posts, a crossbar, ferrules with attached hooks, elastic cables, and on down the line. It furthermore shows the importance of fitness media – whether instructional books or popular magazines like Sandow's *Magazine of Physical Culture* – in spreading awareness about devices of this kind.

As the 1800s gave way to a new century, Sandow's leg machine faced plenty of competition in the 'exerciser' marketplace. The influential educator Dudley Sargent was likewise a proponent of what Carolyn Thomas de la Peña (2003a) refers to as 'mechanized fitness'. Like many of his contemporaries, Sargent devised, among other machines, a resistance-training system that put adjustable weights at one end of a pulley and the fitness trainee at the other. Moreover, through his position at Harvard University, Dudley had a direct line to young people ostensibly in need of re-vitalizing. As de la Peña (2003a) recounts, upon renovating Harvard's Hemenway Gymnasium in the late 1800s, Sargent lined the walls with specially designed machines – 36 in all – for training nearly every part of the body. Indeed, the institutionalizing of fitness in PE, in fitness gyms, and in Young Men's Christian Associations – the last of these increasingly open to exercise as part of the wider 'Muscular Christianity' movement (e.g., see Kidd, 2006) – was important in general in giving fitness technologies a home.

To be sure, not everyone was so keen on new fitness equipment (see Chater 4). But exercise machines came with a promise of vitality – life! – at a time when vitality was allegedly in sore need. Thinking contextually about the physical culture movement, the late 1800s and early 1900s saw much hand-wringing over the 'problems' of industrialization and urbanization. City-bound and sedentary office jobs were becoming more common at the same time that machines were lessening the bodily exertion needed in manual production. A perceived "crisis of physical atrophy" (Churchill, 2008, p. 349) was one outcome of this, as articulated by Dudley Sargent (1906) in his book, *Physical Education*:

> Where once a man's occupation kept him in good health he now has to give what health he has to his occupation and trust to other resources to make up the deficiency. . . .
>   There are thousands of people earning their daily bread who never have occasion in their occupation to use the muscles of the upper part of their body. Few ever have occasion to raise the shoulders or lift the arms above the head; and it is difficult to see how the vital processes

of respiration and circulation can be properly carried on without the frequent use of the muscles about these regions.

(pp. 44–45)

Sargent furthermore opined on how changes in communication and transportation were taking a great toll on the brains and nervous systems of modern Americans. As Roberta Park (2007) recounts, while work was changing, it was still perceived as taxing, just in different ways than in the past. Nervous diseases such as dyspepsia were a mounting concern in particular. In this context, the emergence of devices designed for lifting the arms above the head (to use Sargent's terms) or for bodywork in general is both unsurprising and demonstrative of the perceived link between body and brain. As David Chapman (1994) writes, in Sandow's selling mission in particular, the threats of modernity never faded too far into the distance – for example, daily use of his exerciser machine could supposedly drive away 'Demon Dyspepsia' and 'Insomnia' (Chapman, 1994, p. 115). The irony here, of course, is that, in developing and selling modern equipment, physical culturalists were turning contemporary trends back on themselves: modernizing exercise was a pathway to redressing the ostensible ills of modernization.

Sandow's concern over 'Demon Dyspepsia' is telling of the biopolitics of the physical culture movement. This was a movement about re-vitalizing the individual body, to be sure, but it was also about the overall health of the body politic: exercise was a way of ensuring the survival of the state. As Sargent (1906) wrote in *Physical Education*, vigorous training could break down 'old tissue' and replace it with 'new material', thus energizing the body as a whole. "So it may be argued in regard to the life of a community or nation: it lives in proportion to the activity or destruction of its individual members" (p. 38). In the context of this chapter, the ramifications of this link between individual and state are fourfold.

First, and contra the ancient Greeks, the physical culture movement was about promoting physical activity among women and girls as much as men and boys – it is just that women and girls were compelled towards leanness and sturdiness, and men and boys towards robust muscularity. For Mabel Jenness (1892), author of *Comprehensive Physical Culture*, "The superstitions which taught past generations to regard healthful influences as being unfeminine are being outgrown, and a healthier sentiment is beginning to leaven society" (p. 10). In *Physical Culture for Women*, Belle Gordon (1904) – touted as the 'Champion Woman Bag Puncher of the World' – took a similar view: "There is no reason why men should entirely usurp the field of physical culture" (introduction). At the back of Gordon's text was an advertisement for the Fox Exerciser for Women, yet another mechanized pulley system deemed ideal for home use.

Second, concerns over population health spurred the use of technology in another way: for *measuring* the body. Again, the educator Dudley Sargent offers a telling case in point in this regard, first in that Sargent was indeed keen to measure his students in precise terms and second in that PE in general was a common site for such activity, influenced as it was by the science of anthropometry (Vertinsky, 2003). On one level, Sargent clocked his students' running times, measured the external appearance of their muscles with tape, and used devices like calipers to assess the chest and abdomen. As de la Peña (2003b) writes, however, these initiatives only measured what could be seen on the surface. On another level, Sargent used three machines to 'look' internally: the spirometer, which measured lung capacity as subjects exhaled into a mouthpiece; the similarly inclined manometer, where a quick blast of air from the lungs was registered on a dial; and the dynamometer, generally used to measure strength (de la Peña, 2003b, p. 69). Technologies of this kind in turn lent themselves to *representing* the body in evocative ways. For example, Appendix B of *Sandow on Physical Training* (Adam, 1894) features an 'Anthropometric Chart' compiled by Dudley Sargent comparing Sandow's bodily measurements – from his head breadth to his forearm strength to his lung capacity and far beyond – against statistical norms. As a man who once boasted of lifting and supporting a grand piano forte with eight performers on his chest (Sandow, 1897), Sandow was likely unsurprised to learn that his measurements far outstripped those against whom he was compared.

Third, it is through the link between the individual body and the wider population – between the self and others – that the physical culture movement overlapped with the wider eugenics movement, also prominent at the turn of the century. Eugenics was, broadly speaking, a pseudoscience that "sought to improve society through scientifically controlled breeding" (Vertinsky, 2003, p. 102; also see Daley, 2002; Sandall, 2008) and that more specifically housed a range of sciences under its umbrella: craniometry, phrenology, physiognomy, and anthropometry among them. What often underpinned eugenic thought were fears over the declining stock of the imperial 'races'. Apprehension over industrialization and urbanization in this context reared its head yet again. Now, however, it articulated with fears that immigration was 'polluting' the body politic in ways that posed an existential threat. As Churchill (2008) recounts, in America, public officials such as Theodore Roosevelt, "articulated concerns of race suicide" (p. 369) by implying that immigration from eastern and southern Europe was a risk to the national 'race'. A similar discourse arose in Europe too. In early 1900s France, for example, physiologist Charles Richet warned of 'racial swamping' via the 'wrong kind' of immigration (Tumblety, 2012). For many physical culturalists, muscle was a bulwark against the threat of racial decline. Eugenic thinking easily spiralled together with measurement as well. Physical educator William Sheldon's somatotyping project, for example, was about both measuring young people's bodies on a three-pronged scale and assigning personality profiles to body types of different kinds – physique was destiny (Vertinsky, 2003).

Fourth and finally, and with the earlier three points in mind, the bio-politics of the physical culture movement were such that an ancient theme returned: fitness as a moral pursuit. In a context where personal and population survival were at stake, fit living was easily conceived as a duty for men and women alike. In *Physical Culture for Women*, Belle Gordon (1904) moralized fitness in a way that reflected the pathologizing of obesity in medicine: "Every normal woman has it within her power to develop a perfect and symmetrical figure, and there is absolutely no excuse for the crime of obesity" (introduction; also see Stearns, 2002). In his own sloganeering, strongman Bernarr Macfadden was equally blunt: "Weakness is a crime; don't be a criminal" (cited in Roach, 2008, p. 34).

The fitness boom: fitness as empowerment

The third relevant historical moment in the context of this chapter is the fitness boom of the 1970s and 1980s. Fitness again did not disappear between the turn of the twentieth century and the (approximate) beginning of the first fitness boom. In the spirit of Bernarr Macfadden and Eugene Sandow, for example, Charles Atlas became an icon of physical fitness in the inter-war years, preaching the virtues of meticulous self-care and using his own perfectly shaped frame as evidence that such asceticism works. Atlas, like his fitness forebears, also commodified fitness, in his case by marketing his Dynamic Tension system in the pages of popular publications like comic books. Interestingly enough, Dynamic Tension was apparatus-free, though Atlas faced accusations of disingenuousness based on the idea that he himself relied on exercise machinery in sculpting his Herculean frame (see Reich, 2010; Toon & Golden, 2002). Anxieties over the waning physical fitness of young men and their (lack of) preparedness for war manifested in the Cold War era as well. In America, for instance, President Kennedy wrote in rueful terms of 'soft Americans' in the pages of the magazine *Sports Illustrated* (see Montez de Oca, 2005).

Still, the fitness boom was historically remarkable and has been viewed as successful where earlier Cold War–era fitness interventions failed (Eisenman & Barnett, 1979). The fitness boom is so named in that people and industry alike took greater interest in fitness – consumers surely motivating industry, and vice versa. On the participation front, whilst noting that precise figures on the fitness industry for this time period are difficult to discern, Marc Stern (2008) still paints a picture in broad strokes of growing interest in fitness among the public. By Stern's telling, for example, 1.7 million Americans had fitness club memberships in 1972. This number reached 13 million in 1981, 17.3 million in 1987, and 24.1 million in 1995. Indeed, fitness gyms were evolving. The 'lifestyle gyms' of the 1970s combined features of past-era gyms of many kinds – for example, in bringing together "the gym's traditionally male strength-training activities like boxing and bodybuilding and the exercise salon's female toning exercises of calisthenics, dance and yoga" (Smith Maguire, 2008, p. 72; also see King, 2006).

The growing popularity of jogging and running is yet another indicator that fitness was 'booming'. Patricia Eisenman and Robert Barnett (1979) note that the National Jogging Association was established in America in the late 1960s, the purpose being "to counter lopsided arguments *against* the benefits of jogging as well as to provide sources of motivation for refinement of technique and general enlightenment about jogging" (p. 117, emphasis added). As a measure of the growing popularity of such activity, National Jogging Day saw an increase in participants from 8,000 to 51,000 between 1975 and 1976 alone (Eisenman & Barnett, 1979, p. 117). Over a slightly larger interval, the first New York City marathon had just 126 registrants upon its inaugural event in 1970. By the mid-1980s, organizers reached their limit of 20,000 'official' entrants and had to resort to turning runners away (Radar, 1991, p. 259). Marathon events sprung up in major cities across Europe at this time as well – from Athens (1972) to Berlin (1974) to Paris (1976) to London (1981) and far beyond (Scheerder, Breedveld, & Borgers, 2015). A 'running craze' was underway.

On the industry side, fitness-themed companies such as Nike and Reebok were clear benefactors of, and indeed were drivers of, the 'running craze' and other dimensions of the fitness boom. These two companies in particular were both billion-dollar-a-year businesses by the end of the 1980s, with the lion's share of their profits tied to the footwear market (McGill, 1989). As said in *The New York Times* in 1980, however, other companies had irons in the fitness fire as well:

> Shoe companies aren't the only contestants in the ever-growing running-goods industry. Firms design stopwatches, sweatbands, warmup suits, shorts, cosmetics and health foods especially for runners, and many are doing a runaway business. (Retailers estimate that a dedicated runner spends $200 a year on gear.) In 1977, Hinda Schreiber, a costume designer, fashioned a special brassiere for jogging. The following year, her company, Jogbra Inc., sold 84,000 running bras. By next year, she and her partner expect sales to reach $1 million.
>
> (*The New York Times*, 1980)

As one purveyor of aluminum bicycles said in 1987: "We are riding the whole yuppie fitness boom. . . . Only certain physical types can run marathons – peoples' knees hurt – but fitness is addicting, so people are trying different things" (Fisher, 1987).

Amid this mix of products and services, we find what *New York Magazine* in 1983 called 'space-age' machines (Goldman & Kennedy, 1983, p. 47). Whereas the physical culture movement witnessed a transition from simple tools to mechanical machines, during the fitness boom *electronic* technologies became ever more important.

To be clear, it was not the case that *electricity* was new to the fitness landscape beginning in the 1970s. Rather, the electronic machines of the fitness boom were more sophisticated than the devices that came before them – for example, in supplying customized fitness information via computer technology. A feature article in the magazine *Popular Mechanics* from 1994 is telling in demonstrating the range of technologies of this kind available for purchase (Skorupa, 1994). Among the devices selected for review from a "bewildering number of options" (p. 53) were the following:

- The Lifecycle 6500HR ($1,500 USD), an upright stationary bike equipped with a handlebar-embedded heart rate monitor said to 'effortlessly' register the user's pulse.
- The Bodyguard Quantum Step By Step stair-stepper machine ($1,750), replete with an electronic console for monitoring exercise information, and said to be part of the general trend whereby stair-steppers had moved to the forefront of the home aerobics-machine market.
- The NordicSport Ski 450 ($600), 'cutting-edge' in its graphite composite base and part of the 'explosion' of cross-country ski machines driving the home fitness boom.
- The inelegantly named Precor M8.2E/L ($1,800), fitted with a heart rate monitor as well, and part of the wider trend whereby recumbent (i.e., reclining) stationary bicycles were growing more popular.
- And finally, the Trotter 525 – a device that, with a price tag of $4,200, showed how far the treadmill had come since Oscar Wilde was sentenced to hard labour on its earliest of prototypes.

A feature in *Field and Stream* magazine from 1989 likewise highlighted the benefits of 'electronic trainers': "They're smoother, quieter, more convenient to use than most mechanical systems, and provide a workout customized to your fitness level" (Netherby, 1989, p. 64).

The fitness landscape, then, was growing more complex, both in terms of machines for aiding in the pursuit of fitness and in terms of the *constituent* technologies embedded in new machines. From upright posts, ferrules with attached hooks, elastic cables, and other constituent components of Eugen Sandow's late nineteenth century leg machine, the modern-day Trotter 525 treadmill – even before accounting for its electronic features – included a drive roller, roller pulley, drive belt, motor sheave, speed sensor, electric motor, capacitator, elevation motor, electric choke, and running belt, as per the aforementioned *Popular Mechanics* review (Skorupa, 1994).

Furthermore, in the boom years of the 1970s and 1980s, fitness was also changing in the sense that fitness *media* was evolving – most of all, and in keeping with the electronic theme, in that fitness videos became a popular phenomenon. Certainly, print publications thrived as well. Magazines such as *Self* – the self-professed first women's fitness magazine – *Shape*, *Men's Health*, and *Fitness* were all first published between 1979 and 1992. By 2001, these publications all had paid circulation numbering in the millions (Smith Maguire, 2008, p. 108). The actor Jane Fonda – situating herself in a long line of celebrity fitness entrepreneurs – released five workout books during the 1980s and 1990s. As Louise Mansfield (2011) notes, the first *Jane Fonda's Workout Book* (Fonda, 1981) spent two years at number one on *The New York Times* Best Seller List.

But Fonda is perhaps best remembered for her workout videos. She released 23 of these in the 1980s and 1990s (Mansfield, 2011), facing stiff competition in the process from the likes of Cher and the model Cindy Crawford. Male celebrities such as the rapper Marky Mark, the model Fabio, and the boxer Sugar Ray Leonard tried their hand at exercise videos as well. In one sense, what video offered was the chance to showcase fitness commodities of various kinds. As Margaret MacNeill (1998) writes,

> Cher's workout tape concludes with an advertisement for rubber bands fitness gear by "CherFitness." Similarly [Cindy] Crawford's video contains a Revlon cosmetic advertisement while her trainer Radu advertises himself on his T-shirt. Before the Fonda video workout concludes, the viewer is reminded to "stay tuned for a short review" of her other products. At the end of the Step Aerobic and Abdominal Workout, and extended advertisement for the Fonda library screens like a commercial auto-biography. Every step of Jane's past aerobic history is for sale.
>
> (p. 167)

On another level, though, what video technology offered was symbolic power that outstripped media of other kinds. Cindy Crawford's videos featured a 'bricolage' of Crawford's body parts: "The pageantry of images leaps from colour to black and white, from beach to the warehouse studio, then to the industrial roof top, transferring the audience rapidly through time, space and colours" (MacNeill, 1998, p. 172). Cher, as might be expected, sang along to her own hit song, 'If I Could Turn Back Time' while moving through 'hot dance' sequences in front of her background dancers. Bodies were highly sexualized in texts of this kind. The celebrity body certainly represented an aspirational ideal: slender and toned for women, strong and muscular for men. But the body was also constituted as a *problem* to be dealt with in ongoing fashion. Cher, for example, chastised the fat on her back in one video sequence; Cindy Crawford admitted to working feverishly to attain a 'natural' look. Evidently, the logic in selling fitness in this way was sound. As Smith Maguire (2008) recounts, 15 million exercise videos were sold by 1987.

Thus, whereas electronic fitness machines were novel in offering interactive – if by today's standards, fairly basic – fitness assessments, fitness videos were still didactic and one way in their flow of information. "The messages are directives," say Elizabeth Kagan and Margaret Morse (1988) of Jane Fonda's workout videos, "commands stated without apology, in response to which the viewer is not meant to reply, but to mimic and obey" (p. 171).

In contextualizing this third historical moment, in one sense it is logical that electronic fitness machines and workout videos thrived in the post-war, consumer culture era. This was a time when electronic devices were growing increasingly prominent in general, and not just in fitness. The VCR, for example, was a household staple in the 1980s and beyond (Gray, 1992). As Jane Fonda herself remarked in the early 1990s, hardware was crying out for software – exercise videos helped rationalize the VCR's presence in the home (MacNeill, 1998). Indeed, the technologies of the fitness boom were to a great extent *household* technologies – recognizing, of course, that they could be found in gyms too and that fitness entrepreneurs from earlier eras also sold their exercise equipment as home exercise equipment, as we have seen. This is a point that shall be revisited in Chapter 4.

In another sense, fitness – and certainly fitness technologies too – were implicated in the identity politics of the last decades of the twentieth century. A key message emanating from fitness videos for women was one of *empowerment*. As Mansfield (2011) recounts, Jane Fonda positioned fitness as emancipatory, challenging the idea that women comprise the weaker of the sexes (p. 251). This messaging resonated across advertising in the wider fitness industry. Nike and Reebok, for example, explicitly courted female consumers through marketing campaigns in the 1980s and beyond. Nike's initial forays in this regard were at times ham-fisted – a 1987 ad scolded women for eating like pigs – though by the 1990s the company had become more adept at articulating (and commodifying) feminist discourses of empowerment and corporeal liberation (Lafrance, 1998; also see Cole & Hribar, 1995).

But the commercial version of empowerment was no doubt constrained. In Fonda's case, her fitness texts were apt to promote traditional domestic roles and white, heterosexual femininity, even if they contested the idea that women are inherently weak (Mansfield, 2011). Indeed, female athletes were frequently shown in suggestive poses in popular media, rather than action poses like their male counterparts (also see Carlisle Duncan, 1994; Leath & Lumpkin, 1992). Moreover, as fitness videos and magazines problematized the body, fitness ideals were strengthened anew and arguably were narrowed even further. Excess weight was pathologized, though *over*-musculature in women was often characterized negatively as well. Women could be strong, but not on the level of men. 'Strong is Sexy', boomed the cover of *Shape* magazine in August 1986. Writes Michael Messner (1988), "This caption accompanie[d] a photo of a slightly muscled young bathing-suited woman wielding a seductive smile and a not-too-heavy dumbbell" (p. 204). Body ideals for men were generally inflexible as well. The perception that women were striding towards equality fuelled a backlash against the alleged erosion of male privilege – one that manifested in part through the conflation of masculinity and musculature, aggression, power, and control (e.g., see Jeffords, 1994; White, Young, & Gillett, 1995).

Finally, and in a third sense, fitness technologies cannot be disassociated from the wider late-century shift whereby the politics of lifestyle grew ever more salient. As Benjamin Radar (1991) recounts, in the 1960s, cardiovascular diseases and cancer replaced contagious diseases as the main causes of death. "Simultaneously," he writes, "a growing body of epidemiological evidence indicated that the way persons lived directly affected their health" (p. 258). 'Lifestyle items' – Radar lists obesity, smoking, fat intake, heavy drinking, and the absence of exercise – were deemed to heighten the risk of cardiovascular problems and in some cases cancer too. At the same time, and beyond the issue of health in particular, the rise of lifestyle thinking corresponded with the ascendance of a neoliberal political paradigm – one that, in part, professed the merits of privatized, market-based solutions to social problems in general. By neoliberal logic, the state is to reduce its imprint on society, scaling back public investment where possible to unlock the responsible and creative capacities of people and businesses alike. These were ideal conditions for imagining health as a matter of personal responsibility. Robert Crawford (2006) suggests the relationship worked in the opposite direction too: responsibility for health fuelled the 'common sense' of neoliberalism's essential tenets (p. 410; also see Crawford, 1980).

In this context, lifestyle was construed as a potential problem and *a solution* as well. More to the point, a *fit* lifestyle – achievable perhaps by purchasing fitness apparel, resistance-training equipment, fitness videos, electronic exercise machines for use in the home, and/or a membership to a new lifestyle gym – was a way of enacting healthy, responsible living. As Smith Maguire (2008) writes, the benefits of fitness were, in an obvious sense, written onto the body's surface, albeit in gendered ways. But the benefits of fitness were written onto the internal organs too – a strengthened heart, improved lung capacity, and so on. Indeed, the sciences of physical fitness flourished in the post-war years (see Pronger, 2002). Writing in 1979, Eisenman and Barnett pointed to the work of the exercise physiologist and to emerging forms of instrumentation – biopsies for assessing muscle tissue and electrocardiograms for examining the heart, for example – in assessing the 'internal' benefits of fitness participation. Of most relevance in this regard, however, is the fact that *purchasable* electronic technologies were increasingly delivering insight along these lines as well, giving instant feedback on both activity measures and measures of the body. As said in a 1982 issue of *Popular Mechanics*: "A simple and inexpensive cardiac monitor, like the Heart Alert . . . sounds a beeping tone when set heart rate is reached and a continuous tone at a higher level of effort (usually the maximum desired)" (Nelson, 1982, p. 91). The accompanying image showed a man's torso with a band strapped across it and a wire running from the band to an electronic box. The Heart Alert could be bought at the cost of $110 (USD).

Thus, with lifestyle politics, and with the fitness boom in general, an old theme returned yet again: the moralizing of fitness. Having once been a matter of aligning the human body with that of the gods, and having once hinged on racial survival in the face of 'threats' such as industrialization and immigration, the moral dimension of bodywork now involved 'responsible' self-care as a bulwark against infirmity and as a sign of 'good living' more broadly. In Crawford's (2006) words, "In the 1970s, personal responsibility provided a moral compass for people who came to believe that working on the self by working on the body was regenerative, a way to 'get one's life together'" (p. 408). By Crawford's assessment, the idea of health as a collective responsibility receded into the background (also see Conrad, 1988, 1994; Gillick, 1984). Lifestyle politics brought with them an individualizing logic.

Conclusion: reforming the soul

In *The History of the Tread-mill*, a book published in 1824, author and prison guard James Hardie explained the origins of the treadmill and its use in prison systems in Europe and North America. By Hardie's account, in the state of New York, state prisons were overcrowded, fomenting the need for another structure – the penitentiary – to alleviate this problem. More to the point, prisoners in crowded conditions remained *idle*. "This was a great injury," Hardie (1824) wrote, "not only to the community but likewise to the convicts; as it is one of the principal objects of our system of discipline, to endeavour to reform offenders, by teaching them habits of industry" (p. 13). Hence: the treadmill. As Hardie wrote, "It is [the treadmill's] *monotonous steadiness* and not its *severity*, which constitutes its terror, and frequently, breaks down the obstinate spirit" (p. 18, emphasis in original). Appropriately enough, the word penitentiary is derived from the Latin *paenitentia* – 'penitence'.

The treadmill, in other words, was born as a biopolitical technology. It is in this sense that the plight of Oscar Wilde comes together with the broader narrative of this chapter. Hardie (1824) situated his assessment of the treadmill amid a general discussion of the transition in Western societies away from the politics of death. *The History of the Tread-mill* begins with reference to that centuries-old 'barbarous practice' among European legislators of "endeavour[ing] to lessen the number of crimes, not by the reformation of offenders; but by cutting them off from society, by a shameful and ignominious death," often for trivial offences (Hardie, 1824, p. 9). Evidently, for Hardie, bodywork had a reformative property, both for the body and the soul, and for the benefit of both the individual and the wider population. Moreover, in the quest for 'reformation', technology had a role to play.

At the turn of the twentieth century, biopolitics were not confined to the prison. Existential threats loomed large. Industrialization and urbanization were allegedly weakening the body and brain. As eugenicists would have it, immigration, among other trends, was compromising the racial 'stock' of imperial nations. Under these conditions, exercise in general held the promise of restoring vitality for men and women alike, and thus restoring the nation writ large. Fitness technologies in particular – barbells, dumbbells, Indian clubs, gymnastics wands, and mechanical apparatuses like Eugen Sandow's leg exerciser – were invaluable in the pursuit of fitness ideals. That Wilde was sentenced to hard labour on a mechanical physical activity device near the end of the 1800s was in keeping with the times.

What's more, the fitness boom of the 1970s and 1980s both carried forward and modified many themes and practices from the physical culture movement, and indeed from ancient Greece as well. Barbells, dumbbells, and resistance-training machines could still be found in exercise spaces, though now they had to compete with 'space-age' electronic devices like the Lifecycle 6500HR. The commercialization of fitness and the reimagining of the home as a fitness space – trends that gathered steam in the years of the physical culture movement – only intensified as the fitness industry impressed the virtues of electronic (fit) living in the late 1900s. Moreover, fitness celebrities still held sway. But whereas Eugen Sandow and his contemporaries had to rely on static media like instructional texts and magazines on physical culture in selling bodily ideals and selling their branded fitness commodities, Jane Fonda could take advantage of the dynamism of video.

Most importantly, the fitness boom had a biopolitical dimension as well: fitness was about the self and the wider population both. Yet whereas the physical culture movement to an extent was beholden to the sciences of the eugenics movement (or, at least, a eugenicist interpretation of sciences such as anthropometry), the fitness boom abandoned racial 'survival' as a motivating force and traded instead in the logic of modern life sciences such as epidemiology. The morality of fitness became a question of 'responsibly' staving off chronic disease, especially obesity, as opposed to keeping fit for the sake of racial survival.

The fitness boom also went further in terms of individualizing fitness. To be sure, in the late 1800s, physical culturalists such as Dudley Sargent measured fitness participants in rather sophisticated ways, and in this sense certainly intervened in fitness at an individual level. Yet in sites like PE, bodies were generally treated en masse through activities like military calisthenics (Azzarito, Munro, & Solmon, 2004; Kirk, 1994). Home workout routines were likewise *generic* to a great extent. While Jane Fonda and other fitness celebrities from the late twentieth century were still largely confined to generic messaging, electronic technologies, as said in *Field and Stream* magazine, also had the ability to "provide a workout customized to your fitness level" (Netherby, 1989, p. 64).

As we shall see, the customization of fitness, among other trends, has been pushed even further in recent years. The through-line from ancient Greece to the physical culture movement to the fitness boom leads to the *new* fitness boom as well.

References

Adam, G.M. (1894). *Sandow on physical training: A study in the perfect type of the human form*. New York: J. S. Tait & Sons.

Azzarito, L., Munro, P. & Solmon, M.A. (2004). Unsettling the body: The institutionalization of physical activity at the turn of the 20th century. *Quest, 56*(4), 377–396.

Carlisle Duncan, M. (1994). The politics of women's body images and practices: Foucault, the panopticon, and Shape magazine. *Sport & Social Issues, 18*(1), 48–65.

Chaline, E. (2015). *The temple of perfection: A history of the gym*. London: Reaktion Books.

Chapman, D.L. (1994). *Sandow the magnificent: Eugen Sandow and the beginnings of bodybuilding*. Urbana: University of Illinois Press.

The Chicago Sunday Tribune. (1895). Oscar Wilde on a treadmill: Part 6, 23 June, 42.

Churchill, D.S. (2008). Making broad shoulders: Body-building and physical culture in Chicago 1890–1920. *History of Education Quarterly, 48*(3), 341–370.

Cole, C.L. & Hribar, A. (1995). Celebrity feminism: Nike style post-Fordism, transcendence, and consumer power. *Sociology of Sport Journal, 12*(4), 347–369.

Conrad, P. (1988). Health and fitness at work: A participants' perspective. *Social Science & Medicine, 26*(5), 545–550.

Conrad, P. (1994). Wellness as virtue: Morality and the pursuit of health. *Culture, Medicine and Psychiatry, 18*(3), 385–401.

Crawford, R. (1980). Healthism and the medicalization of everyday life. *International Journal of Health Services, 10*(3), 365–388.

Crawford, R. (2006). Health as a meaningful social practice. *Health, 10*(4), 401–420.

Daley, C. (2002). The strongman of eugenics, Eugen Sandow. *Australian Historical Studies, 33*(120), 233–248.

de la Peña, C. (2003a). Dudley Allen Sargent: Health machines and the energized male body. *Iron Game History, 8*(2), 3–19.

de la Peña, C. (2003b). *The body electric*. New York: New York University Press.

Eisenman, P.A. & Barnett, C.R. (1979). Physical fitness in the 1950s and 1970s: Why did one fail and the other boom? *Quest, 31*(1), 114–122.

Fisher, L.M. (1987). What's new in bicycles: Banking on the yuppie fitness boom. *The New York Times*, Section 3, 21 June, 17.

Fonda, J. (1981). *Jane Fonda's workout book*. London: Allen Lane.

Gillick, M.R. (1984). Health promotion, jogging, and the pursuit of the moral life. *Journal of Health Politics, Policy and Law, 9*(3), 369–387.

Goldman, J. & Kennedy, L. (1983). The last word on health clubs. *New York Magazine*, November, 47–83.

Gordon, B. (1904). *Physical culture for women*. New York City: Richard K. Fox.

Gray, A. (1992). *Video playtime: The gendering of a leisure technology*. New York: Routledge.

Green, H. (1986). *Fit for America: Health, fitness, sport and American society*. Baltimore: The Johns Hopkins University Press.

Hardie, J. (1824). *The history of the tread-mill: Containing an account of its origin, construction, operation, effects as it respects the health and morals of the convicts, with their treatment and diet: Also, a general view of the penitentiary system, with alterations necessary to be introduced into our criminal code, for its improvement*. New York: Printed by Samuel Marks.

Hubbard, T. (2008). Contemporary sport sociology and ancient Greek athletics. *Leisure Studies*, 27(4), 379–393.

Jeffords, S. (1994). *Hard bodies: Hollywood masculinity in the Reagan era*. New Brunswick: Rutgers University Press.

Jenness, M. (1892). *Comprehensive physical culture*. St. Louis: Mecktold & Co.

Kagan, E. & Morse, M. (1988). The body electronic: Aerobic exercise on video: Women's search for empowerment and self-transformation. *TDR*, 32(4), 164–180.

Kidd, B. (2006). Muscular Christianity and value-centred sport: The legacy of Tom Brown in Canada. *The International Journal of the History of Sport*, 23(5), 701–713.

King, S. (2006). *Pink Ribbons Inc.: Breast cancer and the politics of philanthropy*. Minneapolis: University of Minnesota Press.

Kirk, D. (1994). Physical education and regimes of the body. *ANZJS*, 30(2), 165–177.

Kritikos, A., Bekiari, A., Nikitaras, N., Famissis, K. & Sakellariou, K. (2009). Hippocrates counselling with regard to physical exercise, gymnastics, dietetics and health. *Irish Journal of Medical Science*, 178(3), 377–383.

Lafrance, M.R. (1998). Colonizing the feminine: Nike intersections of postfeminism and hyperconsumption. In G. Rail (Ed.), *Sport and postmodern times* (pp. 117–139). Albany: SUNY Press.

Leath, V.M. & Lumpkin, A. (1992). An analysis of sportswomen on the covers and in the feature articles of Women's Sports and Fitness magazine, 1975–1989. *Journal of Sport & Social Issues*, 16(2), 121–126.

Lee, M.M. (2015). *Body, dress, and identity in ancient Greece*. New York: Cambridge University Press.

Macfadden, B. (1915). *Vitality supreme*. New York City: Physical Culture Publishing Co.

MacNeill, M. (1998). Sex, lies, and videotape: The political and cultural economies of celebrity fitness videos. In G. Rail (Ed.), *Sport and postmodern times* (pp. 163–184). Albany: SUNY Press.

Mansfield, L. (2011). 'Sexercise': Working out heterosexuality in Jane Fonda's fitness books. *Leisure Studies*, 30(2), 237–255.

McGill, D.C. (1989). Nike is bounding past Reebok. Retrieved 15 March 2016 from www.nytimes.com/1989/07/11/business/nike-is-bounding-past-reebok.html.

Messner, M. (1988). Sports and male domination: The female athlete as contested ideological terrain. *Sociology of Sport Journal*, 5(3), 197–211.

Montez de Oca, J. (2005). 'As our muscles get softer, our missile race becomes harder': Cultural citizenship and the 'muscle Gap'. *Journal of Historical Sociology*, *18*(3), 145–172.

Nelson, R. (1982). Physical fitness and the machine age. *Polar Mechanics*, May, 91–217.

Netherby, S. (1989). Shape-up system for hunters. *Field & Stream*, July, 64–65.

The New York Times. (1980). Running for the money: Section 6, 26 October, 124.

Park, R.J. (2007). Biological thought, athletics and the formation of a 'man of character': 1830–1900. *The International Journal of the History of Sport*, *24*(12), 1543–1569.

Pronger, B. (2002). *Body fascism: Salvation in the technology of physical fitness*. Toronto: University of Toronto Press.

Radar, B. (1991). The quest for self-sufficiency and the new strenuosity: Reflections on the strenuous life of the 1970s and the 1980s. *Journal of Sport History*, *18*(2), 255–266.

Reich, J. (2010). 'The world's most perfectly developed man': Charles Atlas, physical culture, and the inscription of American masculinity. *Men and Masculinities*, *12*(4), 444–461.

Reid, V.C. (2012). Running wilde: Landscape, the body, and the history of the treadmill. *Critical Survey*, *24*(3), 73–91.

Roach, R. (2008). *Muscle, smoke, and mirrors, Volume 1*. Bloomington: AuthorHouse.

Sandall, R. (2008). Sir Francis Galton and the roots of eugenics. *Sociology*, *45*, 170–176.

Sandow, E. (1897). *Strength and how to obtain it*. London: Gale & Polden, Ltd.

Sargent, D.A. (1906). *Physical education*. Boston: Ginn & Co.

Scheerder, J., Breedveld, K. & Borgers, J. (2015). Who is doing a run with the running boom? The growth and governance of one of Europe's most popular sport activities. In J. Scheerder, K. Breedveld & J. Borgers (Eds.), *Running across Europe: The rise and size of one of the largest sport markets* (pp. 1–27). New York: Palgrave Macmillan.

Shephard, R.J. (2015). *An illustrated history of health and fitness, from pre-history to our post-modern world*. London: Springer.

Skorupa, J. (1994). Heartbeat of America. *Popular Mechanics*, June, 52–117.

Smith Maguire, J. (2008). *Fit for consumption: Sociology and the business of fitness*. New York: Routledge.

Stearns, P. (2002). *Fat history: Bodies and beauty in the modern West*. New York: New York University Press.

Stern, M. (2008). The fitness movement and the fitness center industry, 1960–2000. *Business and Economic History On-Line: Papers Presented at the BHC Annual Meeting*, *6*, 1–26.

Sweet, W.E. (1987). *Sport and recreation in ancient Greece*. Oxford: Oxford University Press.

Todd, J. (2003). The strength builders: A history of barbells, dumbbells and Indian clubs. *The International Journal of the History of Sport*, *20*(1), 65–90.

Toon, E. & Golden, J. (2002). 'Live clean, think clean, and don't go to burlesque shows': Charles Atlas as health advisor. *Journal of the History of Medicine*, *57*, 39–60.

Tumblety, J. (2012). *Remaking the male body: Masculinity and the uses of physical culture in interwar and Vichy France*. Oxford: Oxford University Press.

Vertinsky, P. (2003). Embodying normalcy: Anthropometry and the long arm of William Sheldon's somatotyping project. *Journal of Sport History*, 29(1), 95–133.

White, P., Young, K. & Gillett, J. (1995). Bodywork as a moral imperative: Some critical notes on health and fitness. *Society and Leisure*, 18(1), 159–182.

Chapter 2

A game for everyone

The fitness-technology complex

Looking ahead 20 years, surely no one would have foreseen in 1990 that a sexagenarian actress – someone best known for her depiction of Queen Eliza- beth II, no less – would become a spokesperson for the video game company Nintendo. Gaming, after all, was not just a male-dominated pastime, it was the province of *boys* – or, at least, one might gather as much from the gen- dered make-up of the gaming industry and the gendered themes contained in games themselves. Such was the case, however, that roughly two decades after Nintendo ascended to the forefront of the home video game market, actress Helen Mirren, silver hair and 65 years of life experience in tow, stood aboard the motion-capturing platform for the game Wii Fit Plus, demonstrating its various features at work. For Mirren, the brilliance of Wii Fit Plus lies in its varied exercise offerings. As she says in the ad, exercise is like meeting an old lover: pleasant at first, but soon you remember why you dislike him. The Wii, by contrast, keeps things fresh. It's like having a new lover, daily.

Never could Mirren have imagined herself exercising through a video game console, the actress adds in the commercial, perhaps confirming a sentiment felt by the audience. Doing so inspired feelings of youthfulness (Nintendo Wii UK, 2010; also see Millington, 2016a).

* * * * *

The new fitness boom that is the subject of this book has no single point of origin. Highlighting the release of a single technology as evidence in this regard would overlook that that technology itself was surely 'born' from predecessor devices, from constituent technologies, and from a lengthy plan- ning and development phase as well. Even so, the release of the Nintendo Wii video game console in 2006 stands as an especially important moment in the overall narrative of this book and certainly in the history of fitness as well. The Wii foreshadowed many of the functionalities that would come to define the new fitness boom, as shown in this and subsequent chapters.

Having historicized fitness in Chapter 1, this chapter turns to the con- temporary fitness-technology landscape by examining, in the first instance, Nintendo's very obvious adoption of health and fitness motifs in the mid- 2000s, a corporate strategy crystallized in the company's release of the game

Wii Fit and its sequel games, Wii Fit Plus and Wii Fit U. To this end, the first section of this chapter features a Nintendo case study that traces the release of the Wii back to a twofold crisis plaguing the video game industry and to some extent the wider technology sector in the 1990s and early 2000s. As a console based on an active style of play that is ostensibly conducive to 'everyone', the Wii pushed back against the twin perceptions of video gaming as sedentary and as a pastime for young males alone. In turn, the second half of this chapter is devoted to lessons learned from Nintendo's corporate trajectory from a political economic perspective – with political economy meaning the relationships and interests that underpin industry activity. These lessons pertain to 1) the making of a fitness-technology 'complex', 2) the 'for everyone' discourse evident in technology production and marketing, 3) the human and non-human 'actants' integrated into fitness technologies, and 4) the structural and lived inequalities of manual technology production. The concluding section of this chapter offers reflections on these four overlapping lessons, with attention paid in particular to the hypocrisy of the 'for everyone' logic of the new fitness boom.

Like selling cosmetics to men: the birth of exergaming

As Helen Mirren intimates in pitching Wii Fit Plus to consumers, Wii gaming is generally characterized by its simplicity. On screen, many Wii games, including those that make up the Wii Sports package that was bundled with the console upon its release, have a cartoonish aesthetic. Players oftentimes have the option to create their own 'Mii' avatar as well – again, this being a decidedly caricatured representation of the self. Likewise, gameplay in games such as Wii Bowling (part of the Wii Sports package) is designed to be straightforward and accessible. In their book, *Codename Revolution: The Nintendo Wii Platform*, Steven Jones and George Thiruvathukal (2012) draw a comparison in this regard to video gaming's earlier eras:

> Compared to learning complicated button combinations while controlling analog sticks on a typical game-control pad, using the Wii is remarkably easy. The plain-white rectangular wand shaped like a television remote works by mapping the player's gestures to what's happening in the game world and how the game world is represented on the television screen. In this way, the mimetic interface shifts attention from the game world or what's on the screen to the player's body in physical space, out in the living room.
>
> (p. 3)

The wand in question here is in fact the handheld Wii Remote, a device that is the lynchpin to the Wii's active and embodied style of gaming. The

Remote operates by capturing patterns in movement and relaying these data to a sensor bar located near the television screen. In this regard, the Remote benefits from constituent technologies integrated in production – most of all, an accelerometer that captures movement along the x, y, and z axes, and a gyrosensor designed for capturing rotation. At the same time, in consumption, the Remote is made to integrate seamlessly with the consumer body. As said by Wii developer Akio Ikeda in a production-themed interview series posted by Nintendo online, the Remote can be regarded as an extension of the gamer, as opposed to part of the gaming console (Nintendo, n.d.a). In Bruno Latour's (1999) terms, technologies are folded into the Remote in production; the Remote in turn is folded into the body once this device is actually put to use (see Millington, 2009).

The mimetic capacities of the Wii made this console especially conducive to sporting games, and eventually to fitness as well. To be sure, this was not Nintendo's first foray into the fields of sport and fitness. For example, a 1994 feature in the magazine *Popular Mechanics* on 'Virtual Fitness' reported on an emergent partnership between Life Fitness – makers of the Lifecycle, described in Chapter 2 – and Nintendo of America. The offspring of these companies was the tellingly named Lifecycle Exertainment unit, a blend of the Lifecycle 3500X upright bicycle and Nintendo's popular Super Nintendo Entertainment System console (Skorupa, 1994; also see Bogost, 2007).

It was with the Wii, however, that 'first person' gaming was put front and centre in Nintendo's product catalogue. With the release of Wii Fit in 2007, fitness became an especially prominent theme. Wii Fit introduced a second piece of interactive hardware to go along with the Wii Remote: a rectangular Balance Board reminiscent of a weight scale. In essence, the Balance Board is a controller for the feet (Nintendo, n.d.b). Standing on this platform, gamers can both measure themselves in various ways (see Chapter 3) and partake in training activities ranging from yoga to balance games to strength training to aerobics and beyond – all in the interest, again, of partnering fitness with fun (see Nintendo, 2011). Like the handheld Wii Remote, the Balance Board emerged from a lengthy experimentation phase and from the integration of component parts. "We were developing a piece of hardware that was to be bundled with a piece of software," said producer Takao Sawano in the same interview series referenced earlier. "So if we couldn't keep costs down, we wouldn't be able to sell it." Sawano continues, referencing the Wii's predecessor console, the Nintendo 64:

> Eventually, we hit upon the idea of using the Nintendo 64 Controller. An optical rotary encoder had been built into the 3D stick of the Nintendo 64 Controller, and we decided we could use this encoder in our hardware as well. This was something we'd never attempted before, so it looked

like it would be a lot of fun to work on, and we eventually discovered that the encoder could measure weight to a precision of 100g.

(Nintendo, n.d.c)

Taken together, the Wii Remote and the Wii Fit Balance Board opened the door to a range of health and fitness-themed games, some produced by Nintendo, but many made by third party developers. Wii Fit U, another follow-up to the original game Wii Fit, was released in 2013, and added the Wii U GamePad Controller – an iPad-like tablet that features a video screen, joysticks, control buttons and, once again, a built-in accelerometer and gyroscope (Nintendo, 2016) – to Nintendo's collection of gaming hardware. With Wii Fit U, Nintendo also unveiled the Fit Meter, a wearable tracking device for recording measures such as steps taken, acceleration, and altitude changes. Video gaming suddenly transcended the confines of the home (see Chapter 4).

* * * * *

The question remains: why take such an obvious turn towards health and fitness? Nintendo's 'Exertainment' ventures in the 1980s and 1990s were far from great successes. Surely, there was risk in focusing more intently on fitness, and even greater risk in putting an active style of play at the centre of the video gaming experience in general. It is at this point that corporate motives become relevant. Nintendo was evidently aiming not only to devise a new console and game catalogue but also to change the very image of gaming in the public imagination.

Indeed, in the years before the Wii's release, Nintendo was facing a twofold problem: the gaming market was narrow, and gaming was viewed as obstinately sedentary. To be sure, Nintendo was incredibly successful in the 1980s and 1990s. In the mid-1980s, the company revived a home video game market that had just suffered through the 'Atari Shock'. The company Atari, once at the forefront of the home video game industry, reportedly lost 97% of its annual sales over a period of three years (Coughlan, 2004). In hindsight, Atari's failures have been pinned in large part on overproduction. As Peter Coughlan (2004) recounts, in the early 1980s there were more than 100 independent developers marketing Atari games, and more than 1,000 Atari-compatible games in total. The flood of "cheap, crudely manufactured, and uninspired software" (Coughlan, 2004, p. 5) was a turn-off for consumers – the nadir of the Atari saga coming when millions of Atari game cartridges were literally bulldozed "like the contaminated residues from some unspeakable industrial accident" (Kline, Dyer-Witheford, & de Peuter, 2003, p. 106).

The appeal of Nintendo's gaming systems was surely built in large part on the entertainment value of the company's game offerings. Generally speaking, Nintendo games were (and remain) fast-paced and fun, and were made increasingly so as the landmark 8-bit Nintendo Entertainment System (NES) gave way to more advanced consoles, such as the 16-bit Super NES. Stephen Kline, Nick Dyer-Witheford, and Greig de Peuter (2003) recount how famed game designer Shigeru Miyamoto developed *Super Mario Bros.* with childhood experiences of hiking and serendipitous nature discoveries in mind, the idea being that gamers would 'feel the fun' with their entire bodies (also see Katayama, 1996). At the same time, Nintendo 'solved' the overproduction issue that bedevilled Atari through a patented 'lock-and-key' chip system: the console 'lock' chip could only be opened by a compatible game cartridge 'key'. Thus, Nintendo could still work with production companies such as Electronic Arts, Acclaim, Data East, Konami, Capcom, and Namco, but the lock-and-key system meant Nintendo retained substantial control over the quality of Nintendo-compatible games (Kline, Dyer-Witheford, & de Peuter, 2003). By 1990, Nintendo had sold 17 million NES units in Japan and 30 million units in America, with Japanese customers buying an extra 12 game cartridges on average for every NES purchased and Americans buying an extra 8–9 games. In both countries, an NES system could be found in one in three households (Coughlan, 2004) – one in three!

And yet, even with Nintendo's successes, video gaming suffered a perception problem, which effectively meant Nintendo suffered a perception problem as the industry leader. First, there was the male youth stereotype. To some extent, this was unfair. For example, as Justine Cassell and Henry Jenkins (1998) recount, in the 1990s companies such as HerInteractive and Girl Games explicitly courted and sought to develop a 'girl market' in defiance of gaming industry trends (also see Nooney, 2013). But this is precisely the point: this was done *in defiance* of industry trends. The demographic profile of NES consumers in the year 1990 was telling: 73% male, 66% under the age of 18 (Coughlan, 2004). Moreover, video game companies took steps to appeal to the male youth demographic in particular. In the 1990s, the company Sega emerged on the scene as a competitor to Nintendo, launching its 16-bit Genesis console in combination with an aggressively 'cool' TV advertising campaign aimed at teenage boys – "a demographic targeting underlined by Sega's violent games, such as the notorious heart-ripping version of Mortal Kombat" (Dyer-Witheford, 2001, p. 969). Writing five years before the Wii's release, Nick Dyer-Witheford (2001) characterized video games as 'boy toys'. He noted too how consumption and production were equally gendered:

> [Video games] are played mainly by teenage and preteen males, whose preferences are reflected and reinforced by the industry's concentration on fighting, strategy and sports genres . . . The game industry, conjured into being by technologically adept and culturally militarized men, made games reflecting the interests of its creators, germinating a young male subculture of digital competence and violent preoccupations. The industry then recruited new game developers from this same sub-culture,

replicating its thematic obsessions and its patterns of female exclusion through successive generations.

(p. 971)

The second problem was the gaming-as-sedentary stereotype. 'Today's Kids Turn off Fitness', announced one headline in *The New York Times* in 1990 (Rubenstein, 1990). According to health experts, this 'epidemic of inactivity' was likely down to increased television-viewing time, with video gaming construed as a problem as well. The story was much the same in the scientific literature. A 2004 study of nearly 3,000 children aged 1–12 found that while television actually had no bearing on children's weight status, video games were indeed problematic in this regard (Vandewater, Shim, & Caplovitz, 2004). "This may mean that video game play, but not television use, is indeed displacing the time children spend in more physically demanding pursuits" (p. 83). Gaming in this sense is the true villain in the epidemic of inactivity.

To these problems, the Wii stood as a potential silver bullet. Indeed, these problems dovetailed in the sense that active gaming, or 'exergaming', as it has been called, might at one and the same time both attract new audiences and topple the gamer-as-a-couch-potato cliché. A key goal with the Wii was to be family friendly; achieving this meant paying attention to health, "the very thing that video games were often blamed for ruining" (Jones & Thiruvathukal, 2012, p. 80). Said Nintendo's now-late President and CEO, Satoru Iwata: "We want to appeal to mothers who don't want consoles in their living rooms, and to the elderly and to young women. . . . It's a challenge, like trying to sell cosmetics to men" (cited in Suzuki & Matsuyama, 2006). To quote game designer Shigeru Miyamoto once again: "We thought that the Wii would be a device placed in the living room and be relevant to everyone in the home. . . . The one subject we felt we had to address was health" (cited in Suciu, 2007; also see Nintendo, n.d.d). Deborah Chambers (2012) notes that Nintendo commercials indeed showed the Wii as rightfully placed in the living room, with games played "by all members of a nuclear-style family, by parents, children and even visiting grandparents" (p. 74).

It is with the professed motives of Nintendo developers in mind that Helen Mirren's presence in Wii Fit Plus marketing becomes perfectly logical. As Jones and Thiruvathukal (2012) say, the 'moms' construct is certainly gendered, even sexist. It evokes the long-standing association between women and domestic space. Even so, Mirren's role as a Wii Fit Plus spokesperson is telling of Nintendo's survival strategy in a deeply competitive technology sector: broadening the video game market through the logic of fit and fun technology experience. As Kline, Dyer-Witheford, and de Peuter (2003) observe, the video game industry is one of perpetual innovation: as soon as a new game or console is made, the next one must be devised and must be made even more appealing than the last. For some time, video game companies marched in the direction of verisimilitude with perpetual innovation in mind. And while graphical realism is still an aspiration in the industry, with the Wii, Nintendo turned towards realism in terms of mimicking actual movement in the flesh. Verisimilitude now meant aligning the 'virtual' and the 'real'. This style of gaming was tailor-made for sport and fitness; for Nintendo, this would ideally make gaming appealing to everyone. Said Satoru Iwata in Nintendo's (2006) Annual Report: "Nintendo has implemented a strategy which encourages people around the world to play video games regardless of their age, gender or cultural background. Our goal is to expand the gaming population" (Nintendo, 2006).

Lesson 1: the fitness-technology complex

What lessons can be drawn from the path Nintendo walked from the mid-1980s to the mid-2000s, arriving at a destination where a game like Wii Fit Plus was not only an appropriate fit in Nintendo's product catalogue, but was one of the company's most popular offerings? The remainder of this chapter is devoted to this question, the first lesson being as follows: fitness has become crucial to the technology sector in general.

Nintendo is not the lone technology sector giant to take interest an in fitness in recent years. Apple, Microsoft, and Google have all done the same, in one sense in that these companies house the most prominent online markets for procuring health and fitness apps. As said in Chapter 1, apps are software applications usually designed to fulfil a fairly narrow range of functionalities, leveraging the touch features of mobile technology to provide user-friendly experiences. To take one example of an online app market, Apple's App Store contains a broad range of app categories: books, finance, games, lifestyle, music, news, social networking, and health and fitness, among others. In each of these areas, Apple effectively acts as a gatekeeper between app developers and consumers, subjecting apps to a review process based on criteria such as reliability, performance, and acceptability of content (Apple Inc., 2016a). Reasons for rejecting apps are many, including 'misleading users' (Apple Inc., 2016b). Apple thus maintains a measure of quality control in curating the app marketplace, much as we saw earlier with Nintendo's lock-and-key console/cartridge system for stemming the proliferation of poor quality video games.

In another sense, in recent years the technology sector's biggest players have released fitness technologies of their own. Generally speaking, the model in this regard has been to develop both wearable hardware and activity-tracking software, giving consumers means to record bespoke fitness data and view their results on their smartphone, tablet, or computer. The Microsoft Band, for example, is worn on the wrist and helps users get fit by tracking measures such as heart rate, steps taken, stairs climbed, calories expended, and sleep quality. These measures can then be relayed to the Microsoft Health software platform, allowing for what are said to be personalized and actionable insights (Microsoft, 2016). In a similar vein, Samsung Gear Fit is a wrist-worn activity tracker that can be used in combination with this same company's health and fitness-themed app, S Health. Sony's SmartBand2 goes with the tellingly named Lifelog app. Android Wear goes together with the app Google Fit. Facebook has joined the fray as well, in its case by acquiring the app Moves – an "incredible tool for the millions of people who want to better understand their daily fitness activity" (Albergotti, 2014).

At the same time, the fitness-technology landscape is now profoundly diverse, even with the likes of Apple on the production side of the market. In practice, what the app business model has done is allow a vast array of developers into the fitness 'space'. The mythology of the app era in general is that the app model of service provision effectively democratizes media production: while app market hosts such as Apple take a share of revenue from developers (30% has been reported as the industry standard – Mackenzie, 2012) and, as noted, while Apple takes steps towards policing content, the barriers to entering the fitness marketplace have clearly been lowered since the heyday of Jane Fonda's exercise videos and the (first) fitness boom. The 'gold rush' that characterized the early days of app markets was fuelled by the belief that anyone could cash in, a viral product being more important than an established brand name (Lorinc, Tossell, & el Akkad, 2010; Rowan & Cheshire, 2009). As a case in point, technology reporter Tim Bradshaw (2014) highlights the case of the app 7 Minute Workout. Launched in 2013, and only after developer Stuart Hall searched online to learn what a plank exercise is, 7 Minute Workout had made more than $50,000 (USD) within a year's time. The app allegedly took just six hours to code.

Certainly, hardware production brings costs on another level, though venture capital and crowdfunding present further options for those with significant costs for which to account. As reported by CB Insights in September 2014, the preceding five years had brought more than $1.4B of venture capital investment into private wearable start-ups (CB Insights, 2014). Of course, the category 'wearables' extends beyond the fitness domain and into areas such as brain monitoring. Even so, CB Insights lists Jawbone, Fitbit, and Withings, among other fitness-themed companies, as noteworthy beneficiaries of this investment. Moreover, a report from the technology site TechCrunch from roughly this same point in time highlights the substantial growth in venture funding directed specifically towards fitness tech start-ups in recent years – for example, over $100M (USD) was committed to companies at various stages of development in the third quarter of 2014 alone (Magee, 2014). Crowdfunding can be lucrative as well, though likely not on the same scale as venture capital funding in that it replaces large-scale corporate investment with smaller contributions from individual donors. The wearable device LEO, for example – a leg-worn band that purportedly improves on other fitness wearables by tracking biosignals such as muscle activity and lactic acid levels – earned more than $140,000 (USD) from 605 backers through its crowdfunding campaign on the site Indiegogo (see Indiegogo Inc., 2016).

In the optimistic assessment, venture capital and crowdfunding, much like the app model of service provision, hold the potential to further diversify the supply side of the fitness field, helping innovative ideas come to fruition in the process. The company Peloton, for example, has sought to reimagine indoor cycling in the home (Peloton, 2016). The stationary, Wi-Fi enabled Peloton exercise cycle can be used to livestream spin cycle classes onto a bike-attached computer tablet. "Riding a bike and staring at the wall is stuck in the 1980s," said company co-founder John Foley – which is to say, stuck in the years of the first fitness boom (cited in de la Merced, 2015). That Peloton could have developed this product without the nearly $120M of equity funding it has reportedly received is certainly doubtful (see CrunchBase Inc., 2016). The weightlifting instruction app Spitfire likewise speaks to the ostensible benefits of crowdfunded entrepreneurialism. Earning nearly $17,000 through the site Kickstarter (Kickstarter PBC, 2016), Spitfire marketing puts feminist discourses front and centre:

> Why did we decide to make the app? As long-time athletes, we were upset with the quality of most apps on the market, how they portray women, and the goals they assume we aspire to. Many fitness resources are entirely bodypart-centric and promote 'looks' instead of developing abilities.
>
> (Spitfire Athlete Inc., n.d.)

Spitfire, of course, is just one case it point, but it nonetheless represents the potential – with Dyer-Witheford's (2001) critique of the video game industry's gendered labour force in mind – for heightened diversity in technology production in the age of the new fitness boom.

Thus, the lesson here is highly significant in the overall scope of this book: *to be a technology company at the present moment is to increasingly be a fitness company as well.* Nintendo is evidently just one exemplar of this. Moreover, what further enhances this synergy between fitness and technology is the fact that this equation can also be inverted: *to be a fitness company is increasingly to be a technology company too.* Nike's foray into the wearable fitness-technology market in 2012 via the wrist-worn Nike+ FuelBand is perhaps the best case in point in this regard, though other examples abound. Nike competitor adidas offers the miCoach Fit Smart watch, and pairs this together with the miCoach tracking app. The apparel company Asics recently acquired the exercise-tracking app RunKeeper – and with it, extensive data from the RunKeeper community (see Gibbs, 2016).

Apparel maker Under Armour has been perhaps the most eager among traditional fitness companies to cross over into the digital technology realm. In 2013, Under Armour acquired MapMyFitness, and thus the popular app of the same name, and later acquired the app companies Endomondo and MyFitnessPal as well (Pierce, 2016). Under Armour also recently unveiled the 'Healthbox', a suite of tracking technologies that includes a Wi-Fi enabled scale, a wristband activity tracker, and a heart rate-measuring chest strap – all compatible with the UA Record app and available together at a cost of $400 (USD). Said *Wired* writer David Pierce (2016) in reporting on the release of Under Armour's Healthbox,

> The days of dongles and wristbands and straps are numbered. It won't be long before our fitness trackers are built into our shoes, our shirts, our headphones. Everything will be a fitness tracker, and every fitness company will be a tech company.

This is the making of a fitness-technology complex whereby the fitness and technology sectors are deeply interconnected.

Lesson 2: assembling actants

A second point in connecting Nintendo's plight to the wider fitness-technology landscape pertains to the integration of actants of various kinds in the development of interactive fitness technologies. The term actant is carefully chosen. As per the introduction chapter, an actant is a networked entity – human or otherwise – with the capacity to act; "that is, an entity that other actants in the network recognize, take account of, or are influenced by" (Blok & Jensen, 2011, p. 48). The networks underpinning fitness-technology production are too vast to trace in exhaustive detail here. What is clear and worth highlighting, however, is that both people and ostensibly inanimate 'things' assist in developing the fitness-technology functionalities that are explored in subsequent chapters of this book.

As outlined earlier, Nintendo's story is partially one of technology experts working with component parts of various kinds in building the company's interactive devices. As Nintendo ramped up its fitness mandate with Wii Fit and its sequel games, additional expertise from the field of exercise science was brought into the mix as well (see Nintendo, n.d.e). Helen Mirren's game of choice, Wii Fit Plus, was developed with the help of Dr. Motohiko Miyachi from the National Institute of Health and Nutrition in Japan. Dr. Miyachi provided guidance in particular on 'Wii Fit Plus Routines', the game's pre-devised exercise regimens that are crafted for specific purposes such as losing weight (Nintendo, n.d.f). The making of the Fit Meter – the aforementioned wearable tracking device for the console Wii Fit U – likewise involved experimenting with human participants to ensure the Fit Meter's atmospheric pressure sensor could properly account for altitude changes during physical activity (Nintendo, n.d.g).

The point, in thinking more broadly, is that a combination of human and non-human agencies is a necessary component of technological development in general. Take, for example, the case of Lumo brand products Lumo Back, Lumo Lift, and Lumo Run, all sold by the California-based company Lumo Bodytech Inc. The last of these products, Lumo Run, is a "portable running coach" aimed at improving running gait through various forms of sensor technology – a nine-axis IMU, accelerometer, gyroscope, magnetometer, and barometer among them (Lumo Bodytech Inc., 2016a). The science of Lumo Run is such that these sensors, in combination with algorithmic technology, capture biomechanical data (e.g., on cadence and pelvic tilt) by assessing core bodily movement. "To determine these key metrics for targeted form," consumers are told, "Lumo Run was created in collaboration with leading sports biomechanics experts at Loughborough University in the UK" (Lumo Bodytech Inc., 2016b). Meanwhile, Lumo Back and Lumo Lift are for posture tracking and remediation, the former device comprising a sensor-embedded belt, worn near the waist, the latter product sensing posture by attaching to the front of one's clothing near the neckline. Though Lumo Back has been discontinued in favour of the less intrusive Lift device, Back is nonetheless telling of the potential role not just of exercise science but *data science* in production. In June 2013, a blog entry from Lumo's Data Scientist noted that 15,000,000 pieces of data had been collected from 'LUMObackers' since the year began (Lumo Bodytech Inc., 2016c). In another post from later that same year, it was added that big data of this kind could be put to use in refining the Lumo Back algorithm to be more vigilant in monitoring posture at certain points of the day (Lumo Bodytech Inc., 2016d; also see Millington, 2016b).

The company Fitbit provides another case in point. In 2009, Fitbit provided an interesting and indeed rare look into the development of its movement tracking algorithms in a blog post on the Fitbit promotional website. Fitbit's mode of operation, the post explains, is such that accelerometer technology measures bodily acceleration, generating 'raw data' that is in turn converted through algorithmic technology into information about the user's daily life (e.g., calories burned, steps, and sleep quality). But algorithms themselves must be carefully devised. And so Fitbit has enlisted (human) 'test subjects' in production, having them wear, for example, both the (non-human) Fitbit product and (non-human) 'truth devices' in product testing – the latter providing a measure of things such as gas composition in one's breath, but presumably unmarketable in and of themselves due to their elaborate appearance. This is a process, in other words, of calibrating the Fitbit product to more 'trustworthy' technology (Fitbit Inc., 2015; see Millington, 2016c). Raw data are 'cooked' from the start through the lab-based process of algorithm design (see Gitelman & Jackson, 2013; also see Bowker, 2005).

In all, the point is that while the production side of the fitness realm has grown more diverse in terms of companies involved, per lesson 1, the more specific actants – from data scientists to truth devices to algorithms – involved in developing fitness technologies continues to grow and diversify as well. If it is obvious to say that fitness technologies are made up of constituent components, it is nonetheless an important point, as the actants represented in technology production enable the product functionalities explored in subsequent chapters.

Lesson 3: 'for everyone'

A third lesson from Nintendo's corporate journey pertains to the 'for everyone' discourse referred to earlier. Nintendo has, in recent years, turned rather decisively towards inclusivity in an effort to broaden its consumer base.

Thinking beyond the Wii, the 'for everyone' discourse will be explored in two ways in this book. In Chapter 3, a case will be made that fitness technologies are implicitly 'for everyone' in that everyone's life can allegedly be further optimized. For the sake of this chapter, the argument is that explicitly appealing to different consumer demographics in both production and marketing is indeed a common industry practice. The new fitness boom is for everyone in that seemingly everyone is a sought-after consumer.

The recent emergence of 'brain training', for example, along with brain training technologies that allow for such activity, can be understood in part as a function of changing demographic trends – much as Helen Mirren is an avatar for Nintendo's newfound interest in older consumers. Also known as 'neurobics' (Katz & Rubin, 1999), brain training is based on the science of neuroplasticity: the idea that the brain remains malleable as one ages (see Millington, 2012; Williams, Higgs, & Katz, 2012). Brain training might initially be deemed beyond the fitness realm. Yet, as the term 'training' implies, marketing for brain training technologies often deploys a metaphor of bodily improvement to make brain training intelligible. Like a muscle, the brain can atrophy without proper stimulation, hence the axiom 'use it or lose it' in the selling of products such as HAPPYneuron and Nintendo's Brain Age[2] (Millington, 2012). To be sure, brain training is not just for seniors, though later life has been depicted as a time when the perils of cognitive decline loom especially large. The 'Brain Fitness Coach' HAPPYneuron, for example, is said to be backed by the scientific consensus that brain power is 'boosted' through mental stimulation – use it or lose it. While this is deemed to be true at any age, "retirement often also goes along with less brain stimulation" (HAPPYneuron, 2016). In this regard, brain training technologies are not unlike other lifestyle products and services that capitalize on the growing sentiment that older adults can and should remain active in later life (e.g., see Higgs et al., 2009).

At the other end of the life course spectrum, one finds fitness technologies such as Miiya, a smartwatch similar to the many other wearable fitness trackers now available at the fitness marketplace. Miiya, for example, registers 'active time' throughout the day (see Chapter 3). A key difference, though, is Miiya's target demographic: kids. "Childhood obesity is a global issue," announced a press release promoting the launch of Miiya's $50,000 (USD) Indiegogo crowdfunding campaign. "However, we're yet to see lifestyle technology that can combat this problem effectively" (Miiya, n.d.). In fairness, Miiya is pitched at kids via their parents, who would presumably buy this product in the end. Nonetheless, the 'for kids' design speaks to the manifestation of the wider 'for everyone' discourse. In this same vein, Deborah Lupton and Ben Williamson (2017) describe a range of wearable tracking devices that allow teachers to track children in the gymnasium, on the playing field, and beyond. In all, fitness-technology consumerism knows no bounds at either end of the life course spectrum.

In another sense, the logic of the new fitness boom is evidently such that *particular* technologies can be 'for everyone' as well – or, at least, that the suite of products offered by particular companies can meet the needs of any given consumer. Fitbit's fitness products, for example, are divided into the categories 'Everyday' (for overall health), 'Active' (for making the most of workouts), and 'Performance' (for reaching peak performance). The catchphrase 'Find your fit' intimates that both fitness and consumers are indeed diverse (Fitbit Inc., 2016). For its part, Apple pledges to keep Apple Watch wearers motivated to achieve steady progress, whether the wearer in question is a dedicated athlete or someone fitting 30 minutes of exercise into her daily routine (Apple Inc., 2016c). The imagined market for the company Hexoskin's sensor-infused clothing – pitched as 'wearable body metrics' – likewise runs the gamut from 'regular people' to 'elite athletes' (Carré Technologies Inc., 2016). The Strava app, made for mapping physical activity, among other things, is sold along similar lines: "Not all athletes are the same. Some are young, some are old, some are slim and some are heavyweights – and plenty used to be one and are now the other" (Strava Inc., 2016). Presumably, none of these athletes of varying types are precluded from using Strava technology. In all, the notion that fitness technologies are widely accessible bespeaks an important point: that the demand side of the fitness-technology market, much like the supply side, is imagined as profoundly diverse.

Lesson 4: commodities, fetishized

The picture painted thus far of production in the new fitness boom misses one key element: the manual labour that brings fitness commodities to a tangible state. Nintendo's case again provides telling insight in this regard.

Manual labour has for some time been a contentious matter in the fitness realm. By Michael Donaghu and Richard Barff's (1990) assessment, in the time of the first fitness boom, Nike was representative of a newly emergent production model – one marked by flexibility (e.g., in machinery, labour, and specialization) and by the outsourcing of manual labour to a 'developing periphery', working afar from the 'industrialized core'. Donaghu and Barff (1990) specifically highlight two tiers of Nike subcontracting (or 'production partnerships'): in broad terms, a first tier comprising factories where company products were put together, and a second tier for the production of Nike-specific raw materials. Per Donaghu and Barff's (1990) account, in 1988, all Nike athletic shoes were made outside of the United States in independently owned and operated factories.

As manual labour was outsourced to the Global South, a transnational advocacy network emerged in opposition to Nike's alleged labour malpractices. As George Sage (1999) writes, investigations into Nike subcontractors were carried out by organizations of various kinds, including academic, religious, labour, development, and human rights groups. "To summarize the reports," Sage continues,

> Approximately 75 to 80% of Nike workers were women – mostly under the age of 24 – who routinely put in 10- to 13-hour days, 6 days a week, with forced overtime two to three times per week. A typical worker earned 13 to 20 cents (in U.S. dollars) an hour – between $1.60 and $2.20 per day, which was below their 'minimum physical needs' (MPN), the figure the government as a subsistence level for a single adult worker in these countries.
>
> (p. 209)

The fact that Nike was elsewhere (which is to say, in the Global North) promoting a discourse of empowerment through sport and fitness added a layer of perceived hypocrisy to their overall operations (Knight & Greenberg, 2002).

Nike was thus a lightning rod for criticism. But the point for these purposes goes beyond the fact that a fitness company became synonymous with anti-sweatshop activism. Nike's approach to production was indeed a new approach *in general*.

Enter Nintendo. Earlier, we saw Dyer-Witheford's (2001) criticism of the gendered nature of knowledge production in the making of video games, with male workers designing games for boys. At the same time, on the manual production side of the coin, a largely female labour force in the Global South was put to work in manufacturing microchips for consumer electronics of various kinds – video games included. In a story familiar to Nike observers, Kline, Dyer-Witheford, and de Peuter (2003) point to the case of Maxi-Switch production plants in Mexico's *maquiladora* zones – plants that in the mid-1990s had a combined workforce of roughly 3,000 workers. At the Maxi-Switch Game Boy factory (Game Boy being Nintendo's popular handheld gaming console), teenage girls reportedly worked ten-hour days for $3.50 (USD) a day, working in poorly ventilated areas to the point that workers collapsing on production lines was not uncommon. Such conditions, write Kline, Dyer-Witheford, and de Peuter (2003), were probably not unique.

Concerns over the state of manual production in the technology sector have not dissipated in recent years. Just the opposite: labour conditions at Chinese factories run by Hon Hai Precision – also known as Foxconn – have recently made international news, especially after a series of worker suicides in the year 2010 (see Fuchs, 2014). Foxconn is reportedly the world's tenth largest employer, with a workforce of 1.2 million (Taylor, 2016). Since 2001, the company has been China's leading exporter (Chan, Pun, & Selden, 2013), serving as an electronics contractor for the wider technology sector – most (in)famously for Apple, though for a wide range of other companies too, including Nintendo. The immense scale of Foxconn's operation is surely a reason for its leading position as an industry supplier, though as Jenny Chan, Ngai Pun, and Mark Selden (2013) point out, Foxconn's competitive advantage lies in its ability to remain flexible by reorganizing production lines, staffing, and logistics in short order to meet the downward demand exerted by company clients.

As in the case of Nike years ago, advocacy groups have taken issue with Foxconn labour practices, holding both Foxconn and its client companies to account for a wide range of workplace issues. In October 2010, the organization Students and Scholars Against Corporate Misbehaviour (SACOM, 2010) released a scathing critique of Foxconn's 'military management', drawing from interviews with 100 Foxconn workers to highlight problems such as below-living wage pay, excessive and involuntary overtime, intense pressure from management, and health and safety concerns (e.g., due to chemicals used in production). Jenny Chan (2013) provides further insight in this regard, in one sense by highlighting issues such as Foxconn's Taylorist shop-floor model whereby tasks are routinized down to the second for the sake of meeting production quotas, and in another sense by bringing to light the lived account of Tian Yu, whom Chan says attempted suicide at age 17 while working at a production facility in Longhua. In all, according to SACOM's (2010) report, "Workers at Foxconn are made to work like machines" (p. 10). Chan, Pun, and Selden (2013) note that Foxconn's vaunted flexibility can be a contributing factor in this regard, as the need to reorganize production in short order can send extreme pressure down the production line. For Nintendo's part, in 2012 a company spokesperson admitted that underage workers had been enlisted at a Foxconn production facility, a violation of Nintendo's Corporate Social Responsibility Procurement Guidelines (Ashcraft, 2012; Moore, 2012).

The 'lesson' learned from Nintendo here is that manual labour is part of the supply side of the new fitness boom as well – a point that is, of course, obvious but is also easily overlooked. Indeed, the idea that relations of production are commonly obscured by the fantastical appearance of commodities at the marketplace lies at the heart of Karl Marx's (2007 [1867]) concept of 'commodity fetishism'. For Marx, the table, as a commodity, transcends its ontology as wood as it 'dances' for potential buyers. Or, as David Harvey (2004 [1989]) writes,

> The conditions of labour and life, the sense of joy, anger, or frustration that lie behind the production of commodities, the states of mind of the producers, are all hidden to us as we exchange one object (money) for another (the commodity).
>
> (p. 101)

Evidently, the lesson here too is that workplace relations are relevant to the new fitness boom as well. Certainly, not every fitness-technology company is represented at Foxconn, yet fitness devices are generally reliant on smartphones, tablets, computers, and/or gaming electronics in registering and visualizing fitness data, as explored further in subsequent chapters. It is necessary to stipulate here that companies have not stood still as the public has grown more aware of worker suicides and workplace conditions in general. Apple, for example, conducts audits and special investigations at its facilities (see Apple Inc., 2016d); Nintendo has stressed its scrutiny of suppliers as well (e.g., see Ashcraft, 2012). In taking the long view, though, labour malpractice is a recurring issue in flexible, globalized production. For SACOM (2010), when it comes to devices like smartphones, manual labour is indeed obscured: "We are consuming the blood and tears of workers, a fact hidden from us by fancy advertisements" (p. 4). That these technologies might be used specifically for fitness purposes is an irony surely not lost on those familiar with the case of Nike.

Conclusion: the promise and peril of 'perpetual innovation'

What the above analysis offers in the first instance is an initial sketch of the contemporary fitness-technology landscape. On the production side, we find software developers, engineers of various kinds, exercise and data scientists, crowdfunders, venture capitalists, algorithms and non-human component parts, manual labourers at Foxconn, and beyond. On the consumption side, we find an imagined consumer market that knows no bounds: the new fitness boom is for kids, for Helen Mirren, and for everyone at every fitness level in between. What this chapter also reveals is that the new fitness boom is reflective of the need for perpetual innovation in technology development. In Nintendo's case, this need led the company away from a primary focus on increasingly realistic graphics and towards a simpler, more accessible, and ostensibly healthier style of gameplay. In general, it has led the fitness sector towards technological development and the technology sector towards health and fitness 'solutions' – a fitness-technology complex.

Perpetual innovation and the lessons learned from Nintendo's case should in one sense be cause for cautious optimism. A key theme of this chapter involves the diversifying of the fitness market. One cannot be critical of the highly gendered nature of video game production, content, and consumption that characterized the video game console wars of the 1990s and, at the same time, be completely dismissive of Satoru Iwata's pledge to make gaming a viable pursuit regardless of age, gender, and cultural background. More broadly, and as said earlier, the idea that both crowdfunding and the app marketplace might give upstart companies like Spitfire, purveyors of feminist messaging, the chance to succeed in the fitness realm is certainly a welcome development.

Yet perpetual innovation is a driver of instability and uncertainty as well. For Nintendo, the company's foray into unchartered waters was short-lived, as competitors Microsoft and Sony followed closely on Nintendo's heels with their own motion-tracking devices that are equally conducive to fitness activity – the Xbox Kinect and Playstation Move, respectively. Moreover, Nintendo's attempt to appeal to 'everyone' has brought the difficult challenge of keeping core gamers – those hoping that video game development will continue along its traditional path – satisfied as well (e.g., see Lee, 2013; Kohler, 2011). Pleasing everyone all of the time is no easy task.

More broadly, the flip side of diversification is that the fitness-technology realm grows more and more competitive, to the point that smaller players in fitness can be drowned out amid a sea of options for consumers. For example, as said in the introduction chapter, there are now more than 165,000 health and fitness apps available for download at online app stores. After the early gold rush years of app development, reports have more recently seized on how challenging it is for app companies to stand out in a crowded health and fitness field and how difficult it can be for consumers to navigate this same online space (e.g., see Bradshaw, 2014; Faletski, 2012; Newton, n.d.; Tweedie, 2014). In this sense, the issue of overproduction that befell Atari rears its head again: companies like Apple face the prospect of too many consumer options in their role as gatekeepers between consumers and third party developers. Life is no easier for wearable technology merchants either, or at least the smaller companies among them. GestureLogic Inc., maker of the wearable device LEO, recently filed for bankruptcy protection, despite its aforementioned crowdfunding campaign to raise funds for LEO's development. GestureLogic founder Leonard MacEachern noted that wearable tech companies typically raise funding on the order of $10M, making for stiff competition indeed (Ritchie, 2016).

Of course, the more significant issue in the interminable need to develop and release newer and ever more sophisticated hardware and software lies in the human costs of such activity. The 'for everyone' discourse becomes especially specious in light of reporting on manual production in the technology sector. As outlined recently in *The Guardian*'s Datablog, a Foxconn assembly line employee on a basic salary would take 910 days to earn what is needed to buy the Apple Watch, replete with its fitness-related functionalities (Arnett, 2015) – to say nothing of the harsh working conditions described in scholarly and journalistic accounts. Though perpetual innovation might in one sense inspire optimism, the political economic dimensions of the new fitness boom should beget consternation in equal parts.

References

Albergotti, R. (2014). With app acquisition, Facebook enters fitness tracking market. Retrieved 19 May 2016 from http://blogs.wsj.com/digits/2014/04/24/with-app-acquisition-facebook-enters-fitness-tracking-market/.

Apple Inc. (2016a). App store: App review. Retrieved 19 May 2016 from https://developer.apple.com/app-store/review/.

Apple Inc. (2016b). App store: Common app rejections. Retrieved 19 May 2016 from https://developer.apple.com/app-store/review/rejections/.

Apple Inc. (2016c). Watch: Fitness. Retrieved 19 May 2016 from www.apple.com/uk/watch/fitness/.

Apple Inc. (2016d). Supplier responsibility. Retrieved 10 December 2016 from www.apple.com/supplier-responsibility/.

Arnett, G. (2015). Apple watch: How long would it take a Foxconn worker to earn enough for the most expensive? Retrieved 24 April 2017 from www.theguardian.com/news/datablog/2015/mar/11/how-long-foxconn-worker-earn-luxury-apple-watch.

Ashcraft, B. (2012). The result of Nintendo's investigation into underage Foxconn workers. Retrieved 19 May 2016 from http://kotaku.com/5954397/the-result-of-nintendos-investigation-into-underage-foxconn-workers.

Blok, A. & Jensen, T.E. (2011). *Bruno Latour: Hybrid thoughts in a hybrid world.* London: Routledge.

Bogost, I. (2007). *Persuasive games: The expressive power of videogames.* Cambridge: MIT Press.

Bowker, G.C. (2005). *Memory practices in the sciences.* Cambridge: MIT Press.

Bradshaw, T. (2014). Apps: Growing pains. Retrieved 19 May 2016 from www.ft.com/cms/s/2/d72f0e14-27ab-11e4-be5a-00144feabdc0.html#axzz48AnNhBEH.

Carré Technologies Inc. (2016). About us. Retrieved 19 May 2016 from www.hexoskin.com/pages/about-us.

Cassell, J. & Jenkins, H. (1998). Chess for girls? Feminism and computer games. In J. Cassell & H. Jenkins (Eds.), *From Barbie to Mortal Kombat: Gender and computer games* (pp. 4–46). Cambridge: MIT Press.

CB Insights. (2014). Wearables are hot: More than $1.4B invested since 2009. Retrieved 19 May 2016 from www.cbinsights.com/blog/wearables-industry-venture-capital-2014/.

Chambers, D. (2012). 'Wii play as a family': The rise in family-centred video gaming. *Leisure Studies*, 31(1), 69–82.

Chan, J. (2013). A suicide survivor: The life of a Chinese worker. *New Technology, Work and Employment*, 28(2), 84–99.

Chan, J., Pun, N. & Selden, M. (2013). The politics of global production: Apple, Foxconn and China's new working class. *New Technology, Work and Employment*, 28(2), 100–115.

Coughlan, P.J. (2004). *The golden age of home video games: From the reign of Atari to the rise of Nintendo*. Boston: Harvard Business School.

CrunchBase Inc. (2016). Peloton. Retrieved 19 May 2016 from www.crunchbase.com/organization/peloton-interactive#/entity.

de la Merced, M.J. (2015). Cycling start-up Peloton raises $30 million. Retrieved 19 May 2016 from www.nytimes.com/2015/04/17/business/dealbook/cycling-start-up-peloton-raises-30-million.html?_r=0.

Donaghu, M.T. & Barff, R. (1990). Nike just did it: International subcontracting and flexibility in athletic footwear production. *Regional Studies*, 24(6), 537–552.

Dyer-Witheford, N. (2001). Nintendo capitalism: Enclosures and insurgencies, virtual and terrestrial. *Canadian Journal of Development Studies/Revue canadienne d'études du développement*, 22(4), 965–996.

Faletski, I. (2012). Apple's App Store: An economy for 1 percent of developers. Retrieved 19 May 2016 from www.cnet.com/news/apples-app-store-an-economy-for-1-percent-of-developers/.

Fitbit Inc. (2015). A brief look into how the Fitbit algorithms work. Retrieved 11 May 2015 from http://blog.fitbit.com/a-brief-look-into-how-the-fitbit-algorithms-work/.

Fitbit Inc. (2016). Find your fit. Retrieved 19 May 2016 from www.fitbit.com/uk/compare#.

Fuchs, C. (2014). *Digital labour and Karl Marx*. London: Routledge.

Gibbs, S. (2016). Runkeeper bought by Asics in latest sports brand app acquisition. Retrieved 19 May 2016 from www.theguardian.com/technology/2016/feb/12/runkeeper-asics-sports-brand-app-acquisition.

Gitelman, L. & Jackson, V. (2013). Introduction. In L. Gitelman (Ed.), *'Raw data' is an oxymoron* (pp. 1–14). Cambridge: MIT Press.

HAPPYneuron. (2016). Brain & training: Why train your brain? Retrieved 19 May 2016 from www.happy-neuron.com/brain-and-training/why-train-your-brain.

Harvey, D. (2004 [1989]). *The condition of postmodernity: An enquiry into the origins of cultural change*. Malden: Blackwell Publishing Ltd.

Higgs, P., Leontowitsch, M., Stevenson, F. & Jones, I.R. (2009). Not just old and sick – the 'will to health' in later life. *Ageing & Society*, 29(5), 687–707.

Indiegogo Inc. (2016). LEO: Fitness intelligence. Retrieved 19 May 2016 from www.indiegogo.com/projects/leo-fitness-intelligence#/.

Jones, S.E. & Thiruvathukal, G.K. (2012). *Codename revolution: The Nintendo Wii platform*. Cambridge: MIT Press.

Katayama, O. (1996). *Japanese business: Into the 21st Century*. London: Athlone.

Katz, L. & Rubin, M. (1999). *Keep your brain alive*. New York: Workman.

Kickstarter PBC. (2016). Spitfire Athlete Pro: Strength training app for women. Retrieved 19 May 2016 from www.kickstarter.com/projects/841316976/spitfire-athlete-pro-strength-training-app-for-wom/description.

Kline, S., Dyer-Witheford, N. & de Peuter, G. (2003). *Digital play: The interaction of technology, culture, and marketing*. Kingston: McGill-Queen's Press.

Knight, G. & Greenberg, J. (2002). Promotionalism and subpolitics: Nike and its labor critics. *Management Communication Quarterly*, 15(4), 541–570.

Kohler, C. (2011). Nintendo's game-killing policies alienate biggest fans. Retrieved 21 June 2014 from www.wired.com/2011/06/xenoblade-the-last-story/.

Latour, B. (1999). *Pandora's hope: Essays on the reality of science studies*. Cambridge: Harvard University Press.

Lee, D. (2013). E3: Will console-makers alienate hardcore gamers? Retrieved 21 June 2014 from www.bbc.co.uk/news/technology-22885595.

Lorinc, J., Tossell, I. & el Akkad, O. (2010). The age of the app. Retrieved 19 May 2016 from www.theglobeandmail.com/report-on-business/rob-magazine/the-age-of-the-app/article1510836/?cid=art-rail-economy.

Lumo Bodytech Inc. (2016a). Lumo back. Retrieved 19 May 2016 from www.lumobodytech.com/lumo-back/.

Lumo Bodytech Inc. (2016b). Science. Retrieved 19 May 2016 from www.lumobdytech.com/science-of-lumo-run/.

Lumo Bodytech Inc. (2016c). Enter stage left: The data scientist. Retrieved 19 May 2016 from www.lumobodytech.com/2013/06/enter-stage-left-the-data-scientist/.

Lumo Bodytech Inc. (2016d). The data scientist: The afternoon slump, part 1. Retrieved 19 May 2016 from www.lumobodytech.com/2013/07/the-afternoon-slump-part-1/.

Lupton, D. & Williamson, B. (2017). The datafied child: The dataveillance of children and implications for their rights. *New Media & Society*, 19(5), 780–794.

Mackenzie, T. (2012). App store fees, percentages, and payouts: What developers need to know. Retrieved 19 May 2016 from www.techrepublic.com/blog/software-engineer/app-store-fees-percentages-and-payouts-what-developers-need-to-know/.

Magee, C. (2014). Venture investors get moving with fitness tech. Retrieved 19 May 2016 from http://techcrunch.com/2014/11/10/venture-investors-get-moving-with-fitness-tech/.

Marx, K. (2007 [1867]). *Capital: A critique of political economy, Volume 1, Part 1: The process of capitalist production*. New York: Cosimo, Inc.

Microsoft. (2016). Microsoft band. Retrieved 19 May 2016 from www.microsoft.com/microsoft-band/en-gb.

Miiya. (n.d.). Press release: A smartwatch to fight childhood obesity. Retrieved 19 May 2016 from www.mymiiya.com/press/.

Millington, B. (2009). Wii has never been modern: 'Active' video games and the 'conduct of conduct'. *New Media & Society*, 11(4), 621–640.

Millington, B. (2012). Use it or lose it: Ageing and the politics of brain training. *Leisure Studies*, 31(4), 429–446.

Millington, B. (2016a). Video games and the political and cultural economies of health-entertainment. *Leisure Studies*, 35(6), 739–757.

Millington, B. (2016b). 'Quantify the invisible': Notes toward a future of posture. *Critical Public Health*, 26(4), 405–417.

Millington, B. (2016c). Fit for prosumption: Interactivity and the second fitness boom. *Media, Culture & Society*, 38(8), 1184–1200.

Moore, M. (2012). 14-year-olds employed on Foxconn factory production line. Retrieved 19 May 2016 from www.telegraph.co.uk/news/worldnews/asia/china/9614994/14-year-olds-employed-on-Foxconn-factory-production-line.html.

Newton, C. (n.d.). Life and death in the app store. Retrieved 19 May 2016 from www.theverge.com/2016/3/2/11140928/app-store-economy-apple-android-pixite-bankruptcy.

Nintendo. (n.d.a). Iwata Asks: Wii remote: 1. Taking control back to the drawing board. Retrieved 19 May 2016 from www.nintendo.co.uk/Iwata-Asks/Iwata-Asks-

Wii/Iwata-Asks-Wii-Remote/1-Taking-Control-Back-to-the-Drawing-Board/1-Taking-Control-Back-to-the-Drawing-Board-232376.html.

Nintendo. (n.d.b). Iwata Asks: Wii Fit: 4. A controller for the feet. Retrieved 19 May 2016 from www.nintendo.co.uk/Iwata-Asks/Iwata-Asks-Wii-Fit/Volume-2-The-Wii-Balance-Board/4-A-Controller-for-the-Feet/4-A-Controller-for-the-Feet-237751.html.

Nintendo. (n.d.c). Iwata Asks: Wii Fit: 1. An idea inspired by sumo wrestlers. Retrieved 19 May 2016 from www.nintendo.co.uk/Iwata-Asks/Iwata-Asks-Wii-Fit/Volume-2-The-Wii-Balance-Board/1-An-Idea-Inspired-by-Sumo-Wrestlers/1-An-Idea-Inspired-by-Sumo-Wrestlers-237652.html.

Nintendo. (n.d.d). Iwata Asks: Wii sports: 3. Serving an imaginary ball! Retrieved 19 May 2016 from www.nintendo.co.uk/Iwata-Asks/Iwata-Asks-Wii/Iwata-Asks-Wii-Sports/3-Serving-an-Imaginary-Ball-/3-Serving-an-Imaginary-Ball-217876.html.

Nintendo. (n.d.e). Iwata Asks: Wii Fit Plus: 1. Not a sequel but an enhanced version. Retrieved 19 May 2016 from www.nintendo.co.uk/Iwata-Asks/Iwata-Asks-Wii-Fit-Plus/Interview-with-Shigeru-Miyamoto/1-Not-a-Sequel-but-an-Enhanced-Version/1-Not-a-Sequel-but-an-Enhanced-Version-209472.html.

Nintendo. (n.d.f). Iwata Asks: Wii Fit Plus: 4. Creating an exercise guide for healthy living. Retrieved 19 May 2016 from www.nintendo.co.uk/Iwata-Asks/Iwata-Asks-Wii-Fit-Plus/Interview-with-Dr-Motohiko-Miyachi/4-Creating-an-Exercise-Guide-for-Healthy-Living/4-Creating-an-Exercise-Guide-for-Healthy-Living-229254.html.

Nintendo. (n.d.g). Iwata Asks: Fit meter: 3. Measurement boot camp. Retrieved 19 May 2016 from www.nintendo.co.uk/Iwata-Asks/Iwata-Asks-Fit-Meter/Fit-Meter/3-Measurement-Boot-Camp/3-Measurement-Boot-Camp-839153.html.

Nintendo. (2006). Annual report 2006. Retrieved 19 May 2016, from www.nintendo.com/corp/report/06AnnualReport.pdf.

Nintendo. (2011). Wii Fit™ Plus: What is Wii Fit Plus? Retrieved 19 May 2016 from http://wiifit.com/.

Nintendo. (2016). Wii U™ features. Retrieved 19 May 2016 from www.nintendo.com/wiiu/features.

Nintendo Wii UK. (2010). Helen Mirren Wii Fit Plus. Retrieved 19 May 2016 from www.youtube.com/watch?v=koXke2IrRmg.

Nooney, L. (2013). A pedestal, a table, a love letter: Archaeologies of gender in videogame history. *Game Studies: The International Journal of Computer Game Research*, *13*(2). Retrieved 20 May 2016 from http://gamestudies.org/1302/articles/nooney.

Peloton. (2016). Bike. Retrieved 19 May 2016 from www.pelotoncycle.com/bike.

Pierce, D. (2016). How Under Armour plans to turn your clothes into gadgets. *Wired*. Retrieved 19 May 2016 from www.wired.com/2016/01/under-armour-healthbox/.

Ritchie, H. (2016). Ottawa startup GestureLogic files for bankruptcy protection. Retrieved 19 May 2016 from www.metronews.ca/news/ottawa/2016/03/17/ottawa-start-up-gesturelogic-in-financial-trouble-.html.

Rowan, D. & Cheshire, T. (2009). The app explosion. Retrieved 19 May 2016 from www.wired.co.uk/magazine/archive/2010/02/features/the-app-explosion.

Rubenstein, C. (1990). Today's kids turn off fitness. Retrieved 19 May 2016 from www.nytimes.com/1990/10/07/magazine/today-s-kids-turn-off-fitness.html?pagewanted=1.

SACOM [Students & Scholars against Corporate Misbehaviour]. (2010). Workers as machines: Military management in Foxconn. Retrieved 19 May 2016 from http://sac om.hk/wp-content/uploads/2010/11/report-on-foxconn-workers-as-machines_ sacom.pdf.

Sage, G. (1999). Justice do it! The Nike transnational advocacy network: Organization, collective actions, and outcomes. *Sociology of Sport Journal*, *16*(3), 206–235.

Skorupa, J. (1994). Virtual fitness. *Popular Mechanics*, October, 42–43.

Spitfire Athlete Inc. (n.d.). Press kit. Retrieved 19 May 2016 from http://spitfireath-lete.com/press.

Strava Inc. (2016). Advanced analysis: Premium leaderboards. Retrieved 19 May 2016 from www.strava.com/premium/analysis/filtered-leaderboards.

Suciu, P. (2007). CrunchArcade: Nintendo press conference report.Retrieved 19 May 2016 from http://techcrunch.com/2007/07/11/cruncharcade-nintendo-press-confe rence-report/.

Suzuki, K. & Matsuyama, K. (2006). Nintendo says women, elderly key to Wii game player (Update2). Retrieved 15 September 2012 from www.bloomberg.com/apps/ news?pid=newsarchive&sid=a0kklJ1sNgDI.

Taylor, H. (2016). Who is the world's biggest employer? The answer might not be what you expect. Retrieved 19 May 2016 from www.weforum.org/agenda/2015/06/ worlds-10-biggest-employers/.

Tweedie, S. (2014). Apple's App Store is an ancient and outdated mess – here's what has to change. Retrieved 19 May 2016 from www.businessinsider.com/the-app-store-is-ancient-and-outdated-2014-7?IR=T.

Vandewater, E.A., Shim, M. & Caplovitz, A.G. (2004). Linking obesity and activity level with children's television and video game use. *Journal of Adolescence*, *27*(1), 71–85.

Williams, S.J., Higgs, P. & Katz, S. (2012). Neuroculture, active ageing and the older brain: Problems, promises and prospects. *Sociology of Health and Illness*, *34*(1), 64–78.

Chapter 3

Be your best self

Gamification, optimization, surveillance

The weight scale is not a recent invention. That fixture of household bath-rooms and doctor's offices dates back to the nineteenth century and the invention of the public 'penny scale' in Germany. With a focus on America, where the penny scale arrived in 1885, Kate Crawford, Jessa Lingel, and Tero Karppi (2015) recount how the penny scale quickly became a com-mon feature of public spaces such as groceries and drug stores. The name reflected the cost of use. For a penny, the customer could stand on the penny scale's weighing plate, triggering a spring that in turn moved an arrow on a dial, revealing the customer's weight in pounds, at times to great fanfare. Indeed, some penny scales rang a bell or played popular songs in render-ing their verdict on the user's weight. Games such as Guess-Your-Weight, in which the customer's penny was refunded upon a successful guess, were eventually designed in as well. The point, from a commercial perspective, was to exchange data for money (Crawford, Lingel, & Karppi, 2015). In 1927, penny scales made a net profit of $5 million in America, split between scale distributors and daily operators (Schwartz, 1986).

As Hillel Schwartz (1986) recounts, however, the problem with the penny scale was the modesty of its users. The scale told the truth of the body, but that truth was distorted by layers of clothing that added extra weight. "How far could one disrobe in public?" (Schwartz, 1986, p. 168). The bathroom scale presented a nifty solution to this problem, and thus became common-place in the home in the first decades of the 1900s. Weighing oneself, as Schwartz (1986) writes, became newly intimate, and newly sensual too: it was intimate in that the body could be scrutinized, in the nude, with ease and regularity; it was sensual in that advertisements showed women, now immodestly clothed, looking upon the weight scale's dial.

By no means, then, is the weight scale a recent invention. Even so, the Naked 3D Fitness Tracker takes this time-tested product into the age of the new fitness boom.

Naked is the brainchild of the California-based start-up company Naked Labs, Inc. As hardware, Naked comes in two parts: a full-length, free-standing mirror embedded with camera technology and a wireless turntable reminiscent of the classic bathroom scale. The turntable is in fact a scale in itself, though it also acts as a motorized rotating platform – a lazy Susan actually for Susan – that slowly spins to allow the mirror's embedded sensors to scan the user's body, 360 degrees. As software, Naked comprises an app that displays the user's 3D body model – a highly personalized avatar – while also displaying measures such as weight and volumetric body fat percentage and giving insight into the user's progress in these areas over time. With Naked, then, you can "See your body like never before" (Naked Labs Inc., n.d.a). Carrying forward a long-standing tradition, a promotional video for Naked on the company's homepage begins with a slender woman dropping her bathrobe to the floor as she approaches the Naked mirror and turntable.

*****

Having assessed the political economy of fitness technologies in Chapter 2, this chapter and the one that follows turn their attention to how technologies are actually made to operate. How do fitness technologies work? Or at, least, how are they supposed to work? Chapter 4 shall deal with the issue of mobility, and specifically with how the portable dimensions of fitness technologies, in combination with communication infrastructure that allows for mobile Internet connectivity, has helped fitness activity transcend its institutional confines of old. This chapter considers the interactive dimensions of contemporary fitness experience.

Specifically, and with the case of Naked in mind, this chapter begins by assessing the relationships consumers are asked to forge with fitness-technology hardware and software. Beginning from a physical connection between flesh and technology, a reciprocal relationship emerges whereby technology 'watches' the user and in turn gives the user new means to watch over herself. From there, interactivity extends outwards, as fitness consumers are implored to partake in networks made up fitness experts and like-minded fitness consumers. All of this is potentially fun in that fitness technologies are oftentimes gamified – which is to say, and not unlike the penny scale of old, they often include game-like elements. The potential outcome of such activity is an optimized way of life.

The concluding section of this chapter considers how the fitness technologies of the new fitness boom differentiate themselves from fitness technologies of times' past. The conflation of consumption and production – prosumption – is deemed a particularly noteworthy feature of new fitness devices. The conclusion also identifies points of continuity from past eras, including the lingering salience of healthism and its attendant notion that health is a matter of personal responsibility.

Sensing the human race: towards interactivity

What the Naked 3D Fitness Tracker portends in the first instance is a re-imagined relationship between technology and the consumer body. In

Chapter 2, we saw how technology production necessarily involves the convergence of people and things. Naked, as the product of both constituent
parts and the machinations of human experts such as electrical, mechanical,
and computer vision engineers, is a case in point in this regard as well (see
Naked Labs Inc., n.d.a). But Naked also folds together with the body in consumption. This is an *optic* relationship in the sense that camera technology is
used to assess the body. Of equal importance, it is also a *haptic* relationship
in that a physical connection between body and technology – the foot and
the sensor-enabled Naked turntable – allows Naked to fulfil its prescribed
functionalities.

Such melding of body and machine is now standard operating procedure.
It would seem that, in the new fitness boom, virtually no part of the body's
exterior has been spared in the contemporary quest to merge fitness technology and flesh. Contact points include the following:

- *The wrist and hand.* This is perhaps the primary contact point for fitness
  technologies, as in the case of the seemingly innumerable wrist-worn
  fitness trackers now available for purchase. Smartwatches with fitness
  tracking capacities such as the Apple Watch and Android Wear can be
  placed in this category too. The hand is now a contact point for smart
  jewellery such as Ringly's smart jewellery rings, promoted with the
  promise of effortless step and calorie output tracking (Ringly Inc., 2016).
  Here we might include smart implements as well. As seen in Chapter 2,
  the motion-tracking Wii Remote is said to be an extension of the player
  more so than part of the console.
- *The face and head.* LifeBEAM, with the catchphrase "Sensing the
  Human Race" (LifeBEAM Technologies LTD, n.d.), offers a smart hat
  and smart helmet for cycling, and has also raised more than $400,000
  in a Kickstarter campaign for its biosensing earphones (see Kickstarter
  PBC, 2016). FreeWavz smart earphones come replete with fitness monitoring capacities. The Lumafit ear sensor likewise captures motion and
  heart rate data. Though Google Glass – Google's interactive spectacles –
  has been discontinued in its first iteration, the eyes and the face in general loom nonetheless as sites for technologies to integrate with the
  body going forward.
- *The torso.* Sensor-integrated strap devices such as Under Armour's
  UA Heart Rate – part of the company's Health Box, highlighted in
  Chapter 2 as well – and Wahoo Fitness' TICKR Heart Rate Monitor are
  made to connect with the upper body by wrapping around the chest.
  The company Misfit also presents an interesting case here in the sense
  that its Shine and Shine 2 activity trackers, while wearable on the wrist,
  can also clasp to the body or be worn as pendants to accompany the
  user beyond traditional activity contexts (see Chapter 4). Smart clothing
  presents even more comprehensive coverage of the torso. OMSignal, for

example, offers a biosensing shirt and bra. Athos products are similarly inclined, designed as they are to take electromyography technology out of high performance and clinical contexts and place them in more accessible ones (e.g., see Waxenberg, 2015).

- *The legs and feet.* The Athos product line includes sensor-enabled shorts, in addition to shirts, thus covering the lower body in addition to the torso. LEO, which, as described in the preceding chapter, is unlikely to reach the marketplace, was nonetheless designed to strap onto to the thigh to make use of sensors that (for example) measure electrical activity on the surface of the skin (see Indiegogo Inc., 2016). The product Lechal, meanwhile, comes in the form of sensor-enabled shoes and insoles and is explicitly promoted as the world's first "haptic footwear" (Lechal, 2015). Of course, there is the matter of foot-technology convergence via sensing platforms in the style of Naked's turntable or the Wii Fit Balance Board as well.

Thus, in Mark Andrejevic's (2005a) terms, the new fitness boom presents a reality whereby "nothing comes between me and my CPU" (p. 101). From head to toe, the surface of the body is conceived as a series of contact points for fitness hardware – a trend encapsulated in the claim that smart clothing is effectively a second layer of skin (e.g. see Nosta, 2013). Moreover, on the horizon lies an even closer relationship. Jawbone, known for its activity bands, is said to be developing an ingestible activity sensor, making the stomach an interior contact point for technology (Cipriani, 2015). Before such a product comes to market, (some) consumers might make use of Elvie instead. Elvie is inserted vaginally for the sake of Kegel (i.e., pelvic floor) exercise tracking.

What follows from the question of where technologies attach to the body is the question of what they do once in position. For Andrejevic (2005a), ubiquitous computing via wearable technology is significant in large part in allowing information gathering in an unobtrusive fashion. Haptic relationships are a precursor to interactivity.

As Spiro Kiousis (2002) observes, interactivity is a quality of media consumers as much as any medium itself. This is the basis of Stuart Hall's (1993) famed 'encoding/decoding' conception of the circuit of culture. Those engaging with Jane Fonda's fitness books were indeed implored to take up a productive disposition, "surveying and assessing the topography of Fonda's body; its shape, tone and texture and learning how to develop a capacity to engage in the fitness regime" (Mansfield, 2011, p. 244).

Nonetheless, and in light of the physical interfacing described earlier, interactivity now involves a rather intense form of *reciprocity* – in the first instance as technologies collect data from their users. In broad terms, data are generally collected in two forms: they pertain in one sense to what the body *is*, which is to say its composition; and pertain in another sense to what the body *does* as the user goes about her day. We have seen a good case in point for the former already. Naked, through a combination of optic and haptic technologies, collects data on volumetric body percentage, among other measures of the self. Like Athos smart clothing, then, Naked purportedly takes the data collection functionalities of elaborate machinery – the hydrostatic dunk tank – and makes them available in everyday contexts (Naked Labs Inc., n.d.b). Weight scale-like devices are particularly adept at assessing bodily composition, as they need not rely on user 'confessions' of their own weight to do so. The Garmin Index smart scale features "metrics that matter" such as Body Mass Index (BMI), a weight-to-height measure, body fat percentage, bone mass, and muscle mass (Garmin Ltd., 2016). The game Wii Fit is similarly calibrated, if slightly less advanced, as it puts users through a Body Test upon first use that includes an assessment of BMI (see Nintendo, 2011).

The matter grows more complex as fitness technologies assess the body in action. This can certainly be basic enough: wrist-worn activity bands are generally de facto pedometers, counting movement towards a goal of, say, 10,000 steps in a day. Yet, in the style of the big data movement writ large, fitness metrics are now highly varied: heart rate, calories burned, calories consumed, distance travelled, elevation, acceleration, cadence (e.g., while on a stationary cycle), breathing rate, VO2 max, sleep duration, sleep efficiency, deep sleep, tosses and turns (at night, that is), UV exposure, blood oxygen saturation, pulse volume variations, blood pressure variation, individual anaerobic threshold, bounce, pelvic tilt, pelvic drop, and pelvic rotation – again, the list goes on and altogether makes for the possibility of data in great volume, in addition to great variety. The line between measures of bodily composition and bodily activity is most certainly blurry. The point is that activity metrics are more dynamic than measures of the self. Moreover, the ethos of 'perpetual innovation' described in Chapter 2 suggests that fitness-technology merchants will only seek to expand on existing forms of data collection in the years ahead. The Atlas wristband, for example – a device pitched as a super-tracker – already includes a stable of fitness metrics, such as calories burned, average heart rate, peak heart rate, form score, and workout duration. A number of pending metrics are allegedly on the way, including stability, efficiency, power, rest time, and active time (see Atlas Wearables Inc., 2015).

But this is a *reciprocal* relationship: fitness technologies 'give back' as data are relayed to the consumer. At times, this happens through hardware itself – the Fitbit Flex wristband lights up as one achieves benchmarks towards a daily step-count goal. Yet it is in giving back fitness data that wider technological ecosystems become relevant.

For Henry Jenkins (2006), the notion of convergence is vital to understanding the contemporary technology landscape. Jenkins (2006) is clear in arguing *against* the idea that convergence is strictly a technological process;

it "represents a cultural shift as consumers are encouraged to seek out new information and make connections among dispersed media content" (p. 3). Still, convergence culture comprises, in part, the seamless integration of technological platforms of different kinds. If emergent forms of fitness engagement rest in the first instance on the convergence of flesh and technology, they are subsequently indebted to the ways in which devices of different kinds 'speak' to one another.

The most obvious example here involves how wearable devices such as wristbands and smart clothing relay data to the fitness participant's smartphone – capable as the smartphone is of representing such information in clear and compelling fashion. Take Hexoskin brand smart clothing as a case in point. Hexoskin's biometric catalogue includes a list of now-familiar measures such as heart rate zone, breathing rate, minute ventilation, VO2 max, and cadence (Carré Technologies Inc., 2016). The point worth adding here is that these measures of the self are in turn represented on screen. A measure like minute ventilation (the total volume of air inhaled over 60 seconds) can be displayed in real time via the Hexoskin app, providing immediate insight into one's level of performance. This same metric can be represented in graphical form on the user's online dashboard – perhaps displayed on a laptop or desktop computer. Indeed, graphs and charts are key features of the new fitness boom in general, as they hold the potential to deliver insight into changes in performance or in the body itself over time.

Hexoskin's is not an uncommon arrangement. The Microsoft Health app shows health-related data – "Easy-to-understand graphs chart data that are important to help you understand your current, and changing, fitness levels" (Microsoft, 2016) – on a mobile app and web dashboard. Wahoo Fitness promotes itself as a tech-fitness company whose 'ecosystem' of products reflects Wahoo's dedication not only to capturing and measuring workout data but also to helping people understand what data mean. Every "stride, crank, and squat" is connected to the user's smartphone, tablet, or laptop (Wahoo Fitness, 2016). As Wahoo suggests, representing data is a pathway to making data *meaningful* to consumers. Health and fitness apps like the weight-loss app Lose It! have been shown to include features like performance graphs as well (Millington, 2014a). Nintendo has not sidestepped this trend either: Wii Fit includes a function whereby BMI can be graphed over time. The newer game Wii Fit U allows gamers to sync their Fit Meter (a wearable tracker) to their Wii Fit U profile, in turn gaining access to detailed graphs on matters such as calories burned (Nintendo, 2013).

What's more, all of this is ostensibly fun. If it is not inherently fun, fitness-technology merchants oftentimes attempt to make it so by gamifying fitness consumerism.

Gamification is commonly defined as "the use of game design elements in non-game contexts" (Whitson, 2013; p. 340; also see Ellerbrok, 2011; O'Donnell, 2014; Whitson, 2015). As Cameron Lister et al. (2014) explain, gamification stems from the video gaming realm and includes elements such as self-representation with avatars, three-dimensional environments, narrative context, feedback, rankings, and levels (also see Reeves & Read, 2009). Gamification in *health*, judging from the literature on this specific application, typically involves at least one of six core components: leaderboards, levels, digital rewards, real-world prizes, competitions, and social/peer pressure (also see Miller, Cafazzo, & Seto, 2014). In assessing 261 descriptions for health and fitness apps promoted in Apple's App Store, Lister et al. (2014) conclude that 52.5% of apps contained at least one of these six gamification elements and that 23.8% contained at least three elements or more. The fact that prominent fitness-technology companies such as Fitbit, Jawbone, Apple, and Nintendo have gamified their fitness products to one extent or another is a further sign of the salience of gamification to contemporary fitness-technology experience.

Gamification itself is a form of interactivity: a badge landing on one's Fitbit dashboard commemorating 10,000 steps in a day is effectively a feedback delivery system. Nonetheless, the point for these purposes is that gamification is a potential driving force for the reciprocal relationships described earlier. The app Fitocracy, for example, awards badges for achieving objectives of various kinds – bench pressing a certain weight and reaching swimming distance milestones among them (Miller, Cafazzo, & Seto, 2014). As Aaron Miller, Joseph Cafazzo, and Emily Seto (2014) say of Fitocracy's gamified features: "The achievements are colorful and engaging with different images on each achievement, and there are a sufficient number of badges available to incentivize continued use in motivating the user to attempt to earn them all" (p. 3). As explained on Fitocracy's promotional website, Fitocracy's aim is to make gaming both fun and addictive (Fitocracy Inc., n.d.).

All told, then, the reciprocal relationship described herein is one where technologies are made part of the body and where, at the same time, people are urged to understand themselves in rather technical terms – ideally having fun in the process. This is a relationship of interactivity, but it can equally be characterized as one of *surveillance*. Of course, surveillance has long been a core component of fitness cultures. Fitness participants were implored in the past to scrutinize the likes of Jane Fonda, if only to meticulously deconstruct and assess their own bodies in turn. Foucault's famous conception of panopticism – modelled on Bentham's prison – is one where the presence of the prison guard's gaze could never be confirmed nor disproved, emanating as it did from a darkened central observation tower. The effect, in theory, was such that prisoners needed to assume they were always being watched. Consuming fitness magazines, books, and videos is by no means perfectly analogous to confinement in Bentham's prison. Even so, the argument made in the past has been that a panoptic dimension arises as people are implored to internalize a surveillant gaze, assessing themselves towards the achievement of bodily ideals (e.g., see Carlisle Duncan, 1994; Eskes, Carlisle Duncan, & Miller, 1998; Jette, 2006; Markula, 2001).

But the gaze in the new fitness boom is often more figurative than literal: surveillance often begins as a *haptic* form of surveillance, mediated through the touch. This is no doubt a more intimate form of surveillance (i.e., compared to the panoptic surveillance of fitness magazines), both in the sense that the body's boundaries are breached and in the sense that data extracted from the body are highly personalized in nature. From there, surveillance indeed takes the form of self-surveillance, but in this case, it is 'data doubles' that are to be closely and assiduously watched. That is to say, it is personalized and 'datafied' *representations* of the self that are the subjects of scrutiny. BMI and minute ventilation graphs, among other representational devices, transform perhaps-inscrutable data into an intelligible form.

For Kevin Haggerty and Richard Ericson (2000), surveillance now tends to arise through surveillant assemblages that combine multiple forms of 'watching' and that approach the body less as a single entity to be moulded, punished, or controlled, and more as "a series of discrete signifying flows" (p. 612). Meanwhile, Adriane Ellerbrok (2011) observes how, in contemporary consumer contexts, biometrics and the surveillance mechanisms that generate them are increasingly made playful – for example, when consumer photo-sorting programmes employ the face recognition technology originally used in policing contexts. These ideas come together in the new fitness boom: surveillance arises in multiple modalities and is ostensibly made fun through the process of gamification.

Alone together: towards 'Accountability 2.0'

To describe the functionalities outlined in the above section another way, they are *indicative*, meaning they speak or indicate truths of the body in some form or another, thus making the body meaningful in new ways (see Schwartz, 1986). But fitness technologies are communicative in other ways too – for example, in connecting fitness consumers to like-minded individuals in networked fashion.

First, there is the matter of connecting with fitness experts – the human kind, a caveat that is important for reasons that will soon become apparent. Take Peloton as a case in point. As noted in Chapter 2, Peloton is an exercise bike that at first glance is not unlike the exercise bike of old. But where Peloton improves on its ancestor devices is in its Wi-Fi connectivity: a tablet attached to the front of the bike makes it possible to livestream spin classes – filmed daily from Peloton's New York studio – on a screen directly in front of the user. Peloton, then, is not just about registering personalized metrics such as cadence, resistance, and heart rate, but about connecting fitness participants with remotely located experts.

Other platforms are made for similar purposes. Part of Fitocracy's function, beyond awarding badges, is to connect users to real fitness coaches who in turn deliver personalized nutrition plans and workouts via the Fitocracy app. The competitor app GOQii (pronounced 'go-key') might too have been highlighted in the section earlier in that the GOQii Tracker features metrics such as steps, sleep, and active time. Yet GOQii is also a subscription service featuring a roster of coaches with specializations in areas such as weight management, strength training, and endurance training. Coaches, ideally, can keep users "motivated and accountable" (GOQii, 2016). Powhow, a website and app, connects fitness participants to fitness trainers through tools like video chats as well. Powhow CEO Viva Chu has described this service in rather appropriate terms for this book:

> Back in the VHS or Beta days, you'd have Jane Fonda in your living room, but we're actually trying to take it one step further than that . . . [with Powhow] you can not only work out with them on your own time, but you can also develop a personal relationship with them.
>
> (Sachs, 2015)

In this regard, the indicative dimensions of fitness technologies are paired with both *instructional* and *inspirational* functionalities.

At the same time, and judging from other claims made by fitness-technology merchants, human experts are now *obsolete* in that fitness devices themselves can adopt the role of in-the-flesh experts. In Latour's (1999) terms, this is the act of 'delegating' the once-human activities of coaching and training to anthropomorphized things.

What does it mean to coach or train? If it means recognizing technique, the makers of some fitness devices indeed proclaim that their products tick this box through activity recognition. The aforementioned wrist-worn device Atlas – which comes replete with a 'coaching' mode – can automatically detect what exercise the user is performing and when she switches to a new one. If training or coaching means going further and *assessing* technique, then some technologies evidently have this function designed in as well. The shoe-attachable ambiorun 'pod' device deploys a 'coach algorithm' to assess running form and in turn deliver instructions as exercise unfolds – for example, to decrease or lengthen one's stride (ambiorun UG, n.d.).

Surely, training means to motivate the trainee? The Sensoria Virtual Coach, part of the app that goes with Sensoria smart clothing, is made to cheer its users up and keep them motivated with audio cues – monitoring literally every step at the same time (Sensoria Inc., n.d.a). Perhaps most remarkably, if training means to 'punish' trainees as necessary, some wearable devices serve this purpose too. Lumo Lift, for example, has a feature whereby the Lift wearer is physically buzzed when slouching sets in. That timeless command 'stand up straight!' thus takes on a haptic dimension (Millington, 2016; also see Gilman, 2014). Misfit's Shine 2 tracking device likewise gives subtle vibrations throughout the day to encourage Shine wearers to move, again for the sake of good health. In these ways, discipline, including *automated* discipline, becomes part of the new fitness boom as well, working in partnership with the forms of surveillance listed earlier.

Experts, then, whether residing in-the-flesh somewhere or fully automated, are part of the networks accessible to fitness consumers. With the manifestation of automated expertise, the importance of Chapter 2 is again apparent, as the 'enfolding' of, say, exercise scientists into fitness technologies in production enables the subsequent claim that technologies are fitness experts themselves.

Beyond connecting with experts, a related function involves the ability of fitness technologies to connect consumers to fellow consumers, whether via bespoke platforms or via already-popular social media sites. The new fitness boom both constructs participatory fitness communities and bolsters existing online networks.

To be sure, face-to-face engagement between fitness participants – running groups and exercise classes – has not disappeared. Like in-the-flesh experts, though, face-to-face encounters are increasingly positioned as antiquated, whether in implicit or explicit terms. As said in marketing for the weight-loss app Lose It!, "In-person meetings are so last century" (FitNow Inc., 2016). The fitness communities of *this* century evidently gather online. Strava, for example – an app for mapping athletic activity in combination with GPS-enabled hardware – is explicitly pitched to consumers as a social network for athletes, the idea being that individual Strava users can upload data on (for example) their chosen activity route for others to peruse. Activity databases are thus crowdsourced from below as opposed to delivered by experts from above. Strava's social network is said to number in the millions (Strava Inc., 2016). With Fitstar, an app owned by Fitbit, "You're not working out alone" (FitBit Inc., 2016); friends and family, connected via the app, can offer motivation and support. The weight-loss app Lose It! calls this type of interaction "Accountability 2.0" (FitNow Inc., 2016).

Moreover, in addition to the bespoke platforms offered by brands such as Strava, fitness technologies can be linked to popular social media platforms as well. Technological convergence – the integration of technological platforms of different kinds – rears its head once again. Miller, Cafazzo, and Seto (2014) describe how users can sign up for RunKeeper via Facebook, thereby streamlining the task of inviting (or 'onboarding') Facebook friends into one's fitness network. Fitbit has an exercise sharing option whereby workout results can be communicated through networking sites such as Twitter, Instagram, and again, Facebook. This includes a feature through which quantified workout results can be overlaid onto a user-selected photograph, thus merging multiple forms of representation (FitBit Staff, 2015). Likewise, and as said in a 2012 press release for the app Endomondo, "Users can send real-time pep talks to friends while they are exercising, compete against friends, challenge co-workers and share it all on Facebook or Twitter" (Endomondo, 2012). Endomondo furthermore provides the option for users to have workout data sent straight to Twitter, effectively automating the task of social networking in the process. Gamification features such as leaderboards and in-game challenges (e.g., challenging friends to exercise 'duels') are de facto social networking features too.

The new fitness boom, then, is networked. But it is networked in a particular way. Lee Rainie and Barry Wellman (2012) use the term networked individualism to describe how, in a context where people are emboldened to "seek, scan, sift, sort through, and make sense of more and more information on their own" those so motivated can equally "locate and join forces with others who have sought the same material or shared similar paths of experience and exploration" (p. 280). Online networks leverage the flexible autonomy of their members: with Accountability 2.0, networks can be entered into and left with relative ease and at the networker's will, the trade-off being that relationships are less stable and perhaps then less dependable than they were when Accountability 1.0 was the only option available.

Networking in the ways described earlier – sharing, motivating, challenging one another, and so on – can also be regarded as the enactment of surveillance. This is *lateral* surveillance, a concept Mark Andrejevic (2005b) defines in opposition to more traditional forms of watching: "not the top-down monitoring of employees by employers, citizens by the state, but rather the peer-to-peer surveillance of spouses, friends, and relatives" (p. 481). We might add 'fellow fitness enthusiasts' to this list: if scrutinizing one's own fitness data is understood as a form of self-surveillance, then sharing workout results on social media (or setting up an account to tweet such data automatically) is equally a process of 'watching' and being 'watched'. Albers Albrechtslund (2008) uses the term participatory surveillance to capture the horizontal nature of surveillance as it arises specifically through online social networking. The adjective 'participatory' echoes Jenkins's point that convergence culture is not just a technical phenomenon seen through the integration of technological platforms but one driven by the urge to share. For Albrechtslund (2008), participatory surveillance is playful and productive – something reinforced through the gamification of fitness networks – though Alice Marwick (2012) offers the reminder that even 'flattened' surveillance contexts can be stratified, for example in collapsing different real-life contexts (also see Marwick & Boyd, 2011). The broad point here is that peer-to-peer surveillance is part of the new fitness boom's surveillant assemblage as well, along with haptic and self-surveillance, as described earlier.

Optimization: susceptibility and enhancement

The question remains: to what end? Why partake in technologically mediated fitness activity, potentially subjecting oneself to a surveillant gaze from many different directions in doing so? 'Fun' is one possible response, though fitness merchants set out other reasons as well.

As noted at the outset of this book, Nikolas Rose (2007) contends that the field of biopolitics has become "a space of problems concerning the optimization of life itself" (p. 82). That is to say, biopolitics are not defined, in binary fashion, by the presence of health or the absence of illness. This is a time of optimization, whether in the form of 1) susceptibility, meaning the identification and treatment of the asymptomatic in the interest of preventing future problems, or 2) enhancement, meaning attempts at improving "almost any capacity of the human body or soul" (Rose, 2007, p. 82), often through commercialized forms of intervention. Rose's focus lies with biomedicine, but these two dimensions of the optimization discourse are salient in assessing new fitness technologies as well.

On the one hand, seen through a slightly different lens, fitness-related biometrics can be perceived as *risk* metrics, which is to say they offer quantified insight as to whether the subject is in a worrisome state (Millington, 2014b). The use of the metric BMI in assessing the fitness consumer is perhaps the best case in point. BMI is a weight-to-height ratio (kg/m^2) that dates back to the work of the Belgian scientist Adolphe Quetelet (Eknoyan, 2008). BMI categories are benchmarked against qualitative descriptors: a BMI below 18.5 means a weight status of 'underweight'; 18.5–24.9 means 'normal' or 'healthy' weight, 25.0 to 29.9 means 'overweight', 30 or higher gives a weight status of 'obese'. In a context where the purportedly deleterious effects of overweight and obesity have been widely communicated (see the introduction chapter), gauging one's BMI on the Wii Fit Balance Board or similar device is tantamount to a risk assessment.

'Virtual' coaching is relevant here too, given that devices such as ambiorun (clipped to the shoe), Lumo Run (clipped to the waist), and Sensoria (smart clothing) are all geared towards preventing injuries that stem from poor running form. When Sensoria promises 'smarter' running (Sensoria Inc., n.d.b), the implication, arguably, is that runners are at risk, perhaps in a way that cannot be felt or observed. This implies too that commercial intervention can alleviate the problem at hand. The reason ambiorun's aforementioned coach algorithm is important is its role in injury prevention: "Like a good coach, ambiorun is responsive and coaches to optimize your running style and training intensity based on personal goals to make you run faster, longer and reduce your injury risk" (ambiorun UG, n.d.).

Ultimately, virtually any metric can be construed as a risk metric if, when charted over time, and maybe in graphical form, a negative trend emerges. As Rose (2007) observes, risk is about both the present and future: it is about present-day calculations and interventions into the present in the name of controlling potential futures. To the question, 'To what end?', engaging with fitness technologies becomes a rational activity if quantifying the body can indeed reveal how and to what extent the user might be susceptible to health problems, whether known or unknown from the start.

On the other hand, the second arm of optimization is equally relevant here as well. Beyond attending to specific dimensions of the body (e.g., body fat percentage) and/or fitness activities (e.g., running form), fitness technologies are often accompanied by claims that bespeak grander benefits pertaining to life in general. In the words of technology merchants, fitness technologies are variously promoted as a means for empowering the self, being unstoppable, maximizing health, flourishing, understanding or learning about the body, living longer, achieving more, and, indeed, optimizing health and fitness. Athos smart clothing comes with perhaps the strongest assertion of this kind. Athos products are designed to help build a better human machine (see Mad Apparel Inc., 2015). The corporate aim of Lumo Bodytech Inc. – a company behind both posture and exercise tracking devices – is stated along these lines as well: "We strive to optimize human potential and empower you to be your best self" (Lumo Bodytech Inc., 2016). *Your* best self is a telling claim: optimization follows from customization. This is the manifestation of the 'for everyone' discourse once again (see Chapter 2), though now in the sense that fitness devices, *after purchase*, can be catered to everyone's needs.

The point here is not to suggest that such claims are necessarily misleading. Nor is it to say that such claims are surprising: as per Chapter 1, there is a long history of proclaiming that fitness technologies have wide-ranging benefits. The point, with such claims in mind, is that fitness technologies, having improved fitness experience in the first instance, can ostensibly improve *life itself* in the next. This is a discourse of enhancement. As we shall see in the following chapter, the fact that enhancement is an unceasing quest – as Zygmunt Bauman (2011) says of fitness in general, fitness is a construct with no upper limit – is important when considering how fitness activity is monetized in the time of the new fitness boom.

For Haggerty and Ericson (2000), what sutures surveillant assemblages together is desire, with desire understood not as a yearning or lack, but as an active, positive force – what Nietzsche and later Foucault called a 'will to power'. Haggerty and Ericson (2000) are concerned with desires that energize and help form surveillant assemblages, "including the desires for control, governance, security, profit and entertainment" (p. 609). Some of these desires are certainly relevant to the new fitness boom: gamification makes fitness experience more entertaining; Chapter 4 shall explore the profit motive underlying fitness consumerism. For the time being, however, the above analysis shows how different forms of surveillance – haptic, self-, and lateral surveillance – can be brought together against the backdrop of optimization. With this in mind, fitness technologies take on what Schwartz (1986) refers to as a *subjunctive* dimension – what you could be – to go along with their indicative, inspirational, and instructional capacities.

Conclusion: making life count

Measurement has long had an aspirational component. As Schwartz (1986) says of the transition from penny scales in sites like groceries to bathroom scales in the home:

> The shift from publicity to privacy, from the sociable to the personal, was a semantic shift from the third person to the second person and

from the declarative to the subjunctive – from *what this person weighs to what you should weigh and what you could be.*

(p. 165–66, italics in original)

The intertwining of measurement and means of representation is nothing new either. As weight became a growing source of concern in the early decades of the 1900s, medical departments collaborated with insurance companies in the making of height and weight tables – that is, a system of classification, "differentiating those who fit the ideal from those deemed unfit" (Czerniawski, 2007, p. 289). As Annemarie Mol (2000) famously says of diagnostic devices, such devices do not passively register facts of the body, but rather *create* what counts as normal and abnormal in the first place. This is not unlike Rose's (1999) view of numbers in general: they constitute truths rather than simply inscribing pre-existing realities.

With the earlier analysis in mind, what is remarkable about the new fitness boom is how personalized commercial forms of bodily measurement have become. The fitness device Naked is sold on the basis that it gives new meaning to being nude, given its ability to look beyond the surface of the body. 'Weight' is indeed a blunt instrument for assessing the self, at least when compared to current-day measures.

What is remarkable too is the *extent* to which data can be generated in consumption. In the first fitness boom, consumers were, in the main, just that: consumers. The 'flow' of information was primarily from Jane Fonda, on screen, to the Jane Fonda fan, in the living room – recognizing, as earlier, that technology experience is always interactive to some extent. In the new fitness boom, fitness experience is increasingly a matter of *prosumption*: producing and consuming information at one and the same time.

Indeed, George Ritzer (2014) proclaims prosumption to now be in an intensified phase. On the consumption side – which is to say, on the side of what Ritzer (2014) calls prosumption-as-consumption – prosumption arises through technologies and design features that put people to work: self-serve ATM machines and fuel stations; do-it-yourself supermarket checkout counters; and, most all, Web 2.0, what with user-generated data being Web 2.0's defining feature. On the production side, or prosumption-as-production, as Ritzer calls it, prosumption remains a salient concept in that producing goods and services still demands the investment of time, energy, and resources on workers' and business' behalf.

Thus, Ritzer (2014) echoes Alvin Toffler (1980) in pointing to the contemporary rise of the prosumer. Ritzer (2014) also highlights the growing *automation* of prosumption as an emergent trend. The (human) prosumer grows less important in both production and consumption due to smart machines that operate in ongoing fashion without human intervention. Here Ritzer's diagnosis of the changing shape of prosumption overlaps with Mark Andrejevic and Mark Burdon's (2015) observations on the 'sensor society'. For Andrejevic and Burdon (2015), a key facet of contemporary experience is not just that we produce data in copious amounts, but that data are produced *automatically* through environmental and wearable sensor applications that respond to stimuli and generate processable outputs. Examples abound: "car seats with heart rate monitors, desks with thermal sensors, phones with air quality monitors, tablets that track our moods, and so on" (Andrejevic & Burdon, 2015, p. 22; cf., Kalantar-Zadeh & Wlodarski, 2013). In the 'sensor society', we *generate* more than we participate.

In fitness, we certainly still participate, whether in scrutinizing BMI graphs, searching through Strava's online platform for better routes, or, of course, lifting those bloody dumbbells in the first place. Yet fitness is not just witnessing the conflation of production and consumption in an intensified way – to use the ambiorun pod device as intended is necessarily to produce data – but is increasingly defined by the automation of prosumption as well. Haptic surveillance is one way of describing the process whereby a wrist-worn activity tracker 'watches' and generates (for example) step-count data as the user goes about her day. But this is equally a process of automated data production whereby the role of the (human) fitness participant is largely 'passivized'. The task of producing a step count – imagine literally counting steps taken over the course of a day – is delegated to the (non-human) technology. Even networking can be automated by activating account settings that post workout results directly to social media. It seems only fair that technologies are increasingly positioned as coaches and trainers, given their newfound responsibilities.

The appeal of fitness prosumerism is certainly understandable. In one sense, there is the enticing possibility of transcending one's local circumstances through online networks. The app Argus, promoted with the tagline "Quantify your day-to-day" (Azumio Inc., n.d.), has a 'discover' feature that helps users to find niche health communities. In general, networked individualism is based on the notion that a better network awaits: one's immediate, material circumstances need not be a constraint.

In another sense, in a time of prosumption, fitness experience can allegedly be made meaningful in new ways. Fitness merchants at times use the language of making the user's daily activity 'count', or some variation thereof: iFit, for example, sells its Link bracelet with the tagline, "Make your moves matter" (iFit.com, n.d.). References to counting are clever double *entendres*. The devices in question are, in part, counting devices, but the phrasing might equally be taken to mean that technology reveals otherwise hidden insights. Persuasive technology – "interactive computing systems designed to change people's attitudes and behaviors" (Fogg, 2003, p. 1; also see Bogost, 2007, 2015) – is an increasingly popular concept. The optimist's take on the preceding analysis might well be that subtle reminders like the physical buzz delivered by Lumo Lift when slouching sets in can nudge the user towards better posture, and thus better living in general. As the fitness and technology sectors combine with one another (see Chapter 2), the promise of interactivity in general – that the depersonalizing aspects of mass consumerism can be overcome to rewarding ends (see Andrejevic, 2007) – is a core part of the overall package sold to fitness-technology consumers.

But do fitness technologies "differentiat[e] those who fit the ideal from those deemed unfit," as Amanda Czerniawski (2007, p. 289) says of the height and weight tables first used for insurance purposes in the early 1900s? If it is accepted that bodily measurement inherently constructs ideals, then the proliferation of 1) new means of self-quantification and 2) new means of expressing the outputs of self-quantification are grounds for the proliferation of bodily ideals as well.

Existing critiques of fitness have largely centred on the discursive positioning of the body as a site of moral worth. As said earlier, fitness participants have historically been urged to internalize a surveillant gaze and to concomitantly discipline themselves towards a necessarily gendered bodily ideal. Images of slender-but-toned women and slender-but-muscular men reinforce this same messaging. As Deborah Lupton (2013) observes, underpinning representations of this kind is a vision of the entrepreneurial self, keen to enact responsible forms of self-governance (also see Lupton, 2012, 2014).

The slender ideal has not gone away (e.g., see Dworkin & Wachs, 2009), and certainly lives on as devices like Naked are promoted with the help of sculpted bodies, male and female alike. The point for these purposes is that the subjective self-assessment one might have made in the past – my body vs. the established 'ideal' – can now be partnered with an ostensibly objective, technologically mediated assessment of the body's make-up and its performance. Indeed, objective insights are at times explicitly tethered to descriptors such 'normal' or 'overweight', as in the case of BMI. Marie Öhman et al. (2014), in studying the Wii Fit instructional guide, contend that, beyond BMI categorizations, a shaming discourse exists in Wii Fit when the game suggests (for example) that poorly performing players are weaker than they should be. The couch icon 'awarded' to poorly performing participants on Run-Keeper leaderboards can be construed in a similar way. If optimization exists as a discourse, it necessarily has an inverse side.

At the same time, there is the question of what goes missing from a model of fitness provision that trades in deconstructing, quantifying, and assessing the individual body through different forms of surveillance. Based on a study of 20 popular weight-loss apps in the Google Play app store, Antonio Maturo and Francesca Setiffi (2016) arrive at what are now-familiar conclusions: namely, that the apps use both 'rational' (e.g., quantification and graphical forms of representation) and 'emotional' (e.g., gamification via virtual badges) means to help users deal with the purported risks of obesity. The effect, in Maturo and Setiffi's (2016) assessment, is to obscure determinants of health that extend beyond the self. "The digital frame tends to reinforce the idea that the only reason why people do not lose weight is their motivation or their personal failure to follow through on their behavioural changes" (p. 488). 'Making it count' is clever marketing language, but the point Maturo and Setiffi make is that health and fitness technologies, in their mode of bettering the self, inherently *discount* a range of significant factors that exist beyond the individual's purview, but that bear on health and fitness nonetheless. Matters such as inequality, poverty, or social stratification "can hardly be integrated into a 'gamified' life" (Maturo & Setiffi, 2016, p. 480). The rejoinder here might well be to point to the myriad online networks accessible to fitness consumers. But Accountability 2.0 is telling language: even the notion of community in the new fitness boom is seen through the prism of the active entrepreneurial self.

The point, all told, is that healthism – the notion that healthy living is tantamount to a lifestyle choice (see Chapter 1) – retains its conceptual purchase in this new era of fitness technologies. As Lupton (2013) says in reference to the kinds of technologies described earlier, healthism is now "promoted and promulgated in more detail and more intensely than ever before" (p. 397). Through an assemblage of surveillant modalities, the new fitness boom is about the truth of *your* body specifically, and your body divided into constituent parts and behaviours. Optimized living lurks in the distance, and, indeed, the means to get there can be fun: *amusing* ourselves *to life*. Our wider circumstances recede into the background, if they were ever foregrounded to begin with. The fact that responsible living of this kind now defies spatial constraints is explored in the following chapter.

References

Albrechtslund, A. (2008). Online social networking as participatory surveillance. *First Monday*, 13(3). DOI: 10.5210/fm.v13i3.2142.

ambiorun UG. (n.d.). Retrieved 13 June 2016 from www.ambiorun.com/.

Andrejevic, M. (2005a). Nothing comes between me and my CPU: Smart clothes and 'ubiquitous' computing. *Theory, Culture & Society*, 22(3), 101–119.

Andrejevic, M. (2005b). The work of watching one another: Lateral surveillance, risk, and governance. *Surveillance & Society*, 2(4), 479–497.

Andrejevic, M. (2007). *iSpy: Surveillance and power in the interactive era*. Lawrence: University of Kansas Press.

Andrejevic, M. & Burdon, M. (2015). Defining the sensor society. *Television & New Media*, 16(1), 19–36.

Atlas Wearables Inc. (2015). Retrieved 13 April 2016 from www.atlaswearables. com/.

Azumio Inc. (n.d.). Argus. Retrieved 13 June 2016 from www.azumio.com/s/argus/ index.html.

Bauman, Z. (2011). *Liquid life*. Cambridge: Polity Press.

Bogost, I. (2007). *Persuasive games: The expressive power of videogames*. Cambridge: MIT Press.

Bogost, I. (2015). Why gamification is bullshit. In S. Walz & S. Deterding (Eds.), *The gameful world: Approaches, issues, applications* (pp. 65–79). Boston: MIT Press.

Carlisle Duncan, M. (1994). The politics of women's body images and practices: Foucault, the panopticon, and Shape magazine. *Sport & Social Issues*, *18*(1), 48–65.

Carré Technologies Inc. (2016). Key metrics delivered by Hexoskin. Retrieved 13 June 2016 from www.hexoskin.com/pages/key-metrics-delivered-by-hexoskin.

Cipriani, J. (2015). Jawbone is building a health tracker you can swallow. Retrieved 12 June 2016 from http://fortune.com/2015/10/08/jawbone-ingestible-health-tracker/.

Crawford, K., Lingel, J. & Karppi, T. (2015). Our metrics, ourselves: A hundred years of self-tracking from the weight scale to the wrist wearable device. *European Journal of Cultural Studies*, *18*(4–5), 479–496.

Czerniawski, A.M. (2007). From average to ideal: The evolution of the height and weight table in the United States, 1836–1943. *Social Science History*, *31*(2), 273–296.

Dworkin, S.L. & Wachs, F.L. (2009). *Body panic: Gender, health, and the selling of fitness*. New York: New York University Press.

Eknoyan, G. (2008). Adolphe Quetelet (1796–1874): The average man and indices of obesity. *Nephrology Dialysis Transplantation*, *23*(1), 47–51.

Ellerbrok, A. (2011). Playful biometrics: Controversial technology through the lens of play. *The Sociological Quarterly*, *52*(4), 528–547.

Endomondo. (2012). Press: Endomondo social fitness app named a winner of Microsoft Health Users Group 2012 Innovation Award. Retrieved 13 June 2016 from https://blog.endomondo.com/press/.

Eskes, T.B., Carlisle Duncan, M. & Miller, E.M. (1998). The discourse of empowerment: Foucault, Marcuse, and women's fitness texts. *Journal of Sport & Social Issues*, *22*(3), 317–344.

FitBit Inc. (2016). FitStar: Community. Retrieved 13 June 2016 from http://fitstar.com/community/.

FitBit Staff. (2015). Try the new exercise sharing tool from Fitbit! Retrieved 13 June 2016 from https://blog.fitbit.com/try-the-new-exercise-sharing-tool-from-fitbit/.

FitNow Inc. (2016). How it works. Retrieved 13 June 2016 from www.loseit.com/how-it-works/.

Fitocracy Inc. (n.d.). About us. Retrieved 13 June 2016 from www.fitocracy.com/about-us/.

Fogg, B.F. (2003). *Persuasive technology: Using computers to change what we think and do*. San Francisco: Morgan Kaufmann.

Garmin Ltd. (2016). Vivo fitness. Retrieved 12 June 2016 from http://explore.garmin.com/en-GB/vivo-fitness/.

Gilman, S.L. (2014). 'Stand up straight': Notes toward a history of posture. *Journal of Medical Humanities*, *35*(1), 57–83.

GOQii. (2016). Frequently asked questions: Who is a GOQii coach? Retrieved 13 June 2016 from https://goqiisupport.zendesk.com/hc/en-us.

Haggerty, K.D. & Ericson, R.V. (2000). The surveillant assemblage. *British Journal of Sociology*, *51*(4), 605–622.

Hall, S. (1993). Encoding, decoding. In S. During (Ed.), *The cultural studies reader* (pp. 90–103). London: Routledge.

iFit.com. (n.d.). Link. Retrieved 13 June 2016 from www.ifit.com/link/.

Indiegogo Inc. (2016). LEO: Fitness intelligence. Retrieved 19 May 2016 from www.indiegogo.com/projects/leo-fitness-intelligence#/.

Jenkins, H. (2006). *Convergence culture: Where old and new media collide*. New York: New York University Press.

Jette, S. (2006). 'Fit for Two?': A critical discourse analysis of Oxygen fitness magazine. *Sociology of Sport Journal, 23*(4), 331–351.

Kalantar-Zadeh, K. & Wlodarski, W. (2013). *Sensors: An introductory course*. New York: Springer.

Kickstarter PBC. (2016). Vi. The first true artificial intelligence personal trainer. Retrieved 12 June 2016 from www.kickstarter.com/projects/1050572498/vi-the-first-true-artificial-intelligence-personal.

Kiousis, S. (2002). Interactivity: A concept explication. *New Media & Society, 4*(3), 355–383.

Latour, B. (1999). *Pandora's hope: Essays on the reality of science studies*. Cambridge: Harvard Press.

Lechal. (2015). Index. Retrieved 12 June 2016 from http://lechal.com/index.html.

LifeBEAM Technologies LTD. (n.d.). Sensing the human race. Retrieved 12 June 2016 from http://life-beam.com/#.

Lister, C., West, J.H., Cannon, B., Sax, T. & Brodegard, D. (2014). Just a fad? Gamification in health and fitness apps. *JMIR Serious Games, 2*(2). DOI: http://doi.org/10.2196/games.3413.

Lumo Bodytech Inc. (2016). About us. Retrieved 13 June 2016 from www.lumobodytech.com/about/.

Lupton, D. (2012). M-health and health promotion: The digital cyborg and surveillance society. *Social Theory & Health, 10*(3), 229–244.

Lupton, D. (2013). Quantifying the body: Monitoring and measuring health in the age of mHealth technologies. *Critical Public Health, 23*(4), 393–403.

Lupton, D. (2014). Apps as artefacts: Towards a critical perspective on mobile health and medical apps. *Societies, 4*(4), 606–622.

Mad Apparel Inc. (2015). Retrieved 13 June 2016 from www.liveathos.com/.

Mansfield, L. (2011). 'Sexercise': Working out heterosexuality in Jane Fonda's fitness books. *Leisure Studies, 30*(2), 237–255.

Markula, P. (2001). Beyond the perfect body: Women's body image distortion in fitness magazine discourse. *Journal of Sport & Social Issues, 25*(2), 158–179.

Marwick, A.E. (2012). The public domain: Social surveillance in everyday life. *Surveillance & Society, 9*(4), 378–393.

Marwick, A.E. & Boyd, D. (2011). I tweet honestly, I tweet passionately: Twitter users, context collapse, and the imagined audience. *New Media & Society, 13*(1), 114–133.

Maturo, A. & Setiffi, F. (2016). The gamification of risk: How health apps foster self-confidence and why this is not enough. *Health, Risk & Society, 17*(7–8), 477–494.

Microsoft. (2016). Microsoft health. Retrieved 13 June 2016 from www.microsoft.com/microsoft-health/en-gb.

Miller, A.S., Cafazzo, J.A. & Seto, E.S. (2014). A game plan: Gamification design principles in mHealth applications for chronic disease management. *Health Informatics Journal, 22*(2), 184–193.

Millington, B. (2014a). Smartphone apps and the mobile privatization of health and fitness. *Critical Studies in Media Communication, 31*(5), 479–493.

Millington, B. (2014b). Amusing ourselves to life: Fitness consumerism and the birth of bio-games. *Journal of Sport and Social Issues*, *38*(6), 491–508.

Millington, B. (2016). 'Quantify the invisible': Notes toward a future of posture. *Critical Public Health*, *26*(4), 405–417.

Mol, A. (2000). What diagnostic devices do: The case of blood sugar measurement. *Theoretical Measurement and Bioethics*, *21*(1), 9–22.

Naked Labs Inc. (n.d.a). Naked 3D fitness tracker. Retrieved 12 June 2016 from https://naked.fit.

Naked Labs Inc. (n.d.b). Frequently asked questions. Retrieved 12 June 2016 from https://naked.fit/faq/.

Nintendo. (2011). Wii Fit™ Plus: What is Wii Fit Plus? Retrieved 19 May 2016 from http://wiifit.com/.

Nintendo. (2013). Wii Fit™ U: Fit meter. Retrieved 19 May 2016 from http://wiifitu.nintendo.com/fit-meter/.

Nosta, J. (2013). Hexoskin: A second skin for the quantified athlete and maybe even you! Retrieved 12 June 2016 from www.forbes.com/sites/johnnosta/2013/06/30/hexoskin-a-second-skin-for-the-quantified-athlete-and-maybe-even-you/#1cd4f7df40a7.

O'Donnell, C. (2014). Getting played: Gamification, bullshit, and the rise of algorithmic surveillance. *Surveillance & Society*, *12*(3), 349–359.

Öhman, M., Almqvist, J., Meckbach, J. & Quennerstedt, M. (2014). Competing for ideal bodies: A study of exergames used as teaching aids in schools. *Critical Public Health*, *24*(2), 196–209.

Rainie, L. & Wellman, B. (2012). *Networked: The new social operating system*. Cambridge: MIT Press.

Reeves, B. & Read, J.L. (2009). *Total engagement: Using games and virtual worlds to change the way people work and businesses compete*. Boston: Harvard Business School Publishing.

Ringly Inc. (2016). Aries: Step tracking. Retrieved 12 June 2016 from https://ringly.com/aries.

Ritzer, G. (2014). Automating prosumption: The decline of the prosumer and the rise of the prosuming machines. *Journal of Consumer Culture*, *15*(3), 407–424.

Rose, N. (1999). *Powers of freedom: Reframing political thought*. Cambridge: Cambridge University Press.

Rose, N. (2007). *The politics of life itself: Biomedicine, power, and subjectivity in the twenty-first century*. Princeton: Princeton University Press.

Sachs, R. (2015). Beyond Jane Fonda tapes: Home workouts go virtual. Retrieved 13 June 2016 from www.npr.org/sections/alltechconsidered/2015/08/26/434594084/bey-ond-jane-fonda-tapes-home-workouts-go-virtual.

Schwartz, H. (1986). *Never satisfied: A cultural history of diets, fantasies and fat*. New York: The Free Press.

Sensoria Inc. (n.d.a). Run. Retrieved 13 June 2016 from www.sensoriafitness.com/run.

Sensoria Inc. (n.d.b). Retrieved 13 June 2016 from www.sensoriafitness.com/.

Strava Inc. (2016). About us. Retrieved 13 June 2016 from www.strava.com/about.

Toffler, A. (1980). *The third wave*. New York: William Morrow.

Wahoo Fitness. (2016). About us. Retrieved 13 June 2016 from http://uk.wahoofitness.com/about-us.

Waxenberg, J. (2015). The Athos blog: Take your training to the next level with muscle effort training. Retrieved 12 June 2016 from www.liveathos.com/blog/fitness/take-your-training-to-the-next-level-with-muscle-effort-training-2-208.

Whitson, J.R. (2013). Gaming the quantified self. *Surveillance & Society*, *11*(1–2), 163–176.

Whitson, J.R. (2015). Foucault's Fitbit: Governance and gamification. In S. Walz & S. Deterding (Eds.), *The gameful world: Approaches, issues, applications* (pp. 339–358). Boston: MIT Press.

Chapter 4

Anywhere, anytime
Fitness technology and mobile privatization

Charles Wesley Emerson's legacy will forever be tied to his eponymous college. In 1891, the Boston Conservatory of Elocution and Dramatic Art became Emerson College of Oratory. In the context of this book, however, Emerson is relevant as a devoted spokesperson for physical culture. Among Emerson's contributions in this regard were the books *Physical Culture* (1891) and *Expressive Physical Culture* (1900), the latter titled *Philosophy of Gesture* as well. In *Expressive Physical Culture*, Emerson (1900) shows his religious grounding by starting his excursus from the premise that the universe is the externalization of Divine Being and that the human body is a medium through which divinity expresses itself outwardly. Bodily training was necessary in the sense that "a body is beautiful in the ratio that it expresses the noblest states of mind" (Emerson, 1900, p. 48). Physical culture was thus a means for obtaining health and strength and a way of revealing refinement and culture – hence Emerson's general approach and, more specifically, the qualifier 'expressive' in the title of his book from the year 1900.

For the sake of *this* chapter, Emerson is relevant for a more specific reason: his view of where and when physical activity should take place. The answer to the 'when' question in one sense was simple: at every age. But 'when' also came together with 'where' in that exercise should be repeated daily, regardless of location. In this latter sense, Emerson's natural approach was of great merit:

> Our system requires no apparatus; it calls for no room especially prepared for exercises; it makes no further demands for a special costume than that the clothing worn during exercise, must be loose and free. It needs neither clubs, rings, weights, dumb-bells, parallel bars, nor any of the things to be found in a well-furnished gymnasium. I am not an antagonist of these things. They are doing good in their place and time, *but we cannot carry gymnasiums about with us.*
> (Emerson, 1891, p. 19, emphasis added)

In a context where simple tools like dumbbells were increasingly complemented by simple machines like pulley-enabled weightlifting apparatuses (see Chapter 1), Emerson's expressive physical culture was valuable in that it transcended institutional confines.

This chapter is about the idea that, at the current moment, the gym can indeed be carried about with us as our days unfold.

* * * * *

The term 'mHealth' (mobile Health) has earned cachet in academia and beyond in recent years. In 2009, for example, the United Nations Foundation launched the mHealth Alliance, an initiative "dedicated to enabling quality health at the farthest reaches of wireless networks" (United Nations Foundation, 2012). MHealth runs the gamut from proper medical devices – 'smart' glucose monitors for those with diabetes, for instance – to the fitness technologies described to this point in this book. Indeed, as said before, the analysis presented in Chapter 4 of this book in many ways accompanies the ideas featured in Chapter 3. The central point of Chapter 3 was to explore how fitness technologies, in the idealized view of those developing and/or promoting them, are made to work. This chapter considers the *portable* dimension of fitness-technology experience. Once fitness is made wearable, the functionalities of fitness technologies are potentially accessible anytime and anywhere.

The analysis that follows is divided into two substantive parts. The first section focuses on a seemingly inarguable point: that the fitness landscape is now characterized by the 'frictionless' movement of both people and data. This first section draws from Raymond Williams's (2004 [1974]) influential notion of mobile privatization and from work by those who have effectively sought to update this concept in light of recent changes in the nature of telecommunication. The second section, however, casts doubt on the seemingly imminent death of enclosure. It does so first by pointing to corporate wellness programs as exemplars of the recentralizing of data and second by considering the general practice of expropriating consumer data for commercial purposes. The concluding section of the analysis shows the interwoven nature of Chapters 3 and 4, circling back as it does to the preceding chapter to consider issues such as prosumption and consumer responsibility in relation to the mobile dimensions of our current era of Fitness 2.0.

Mobile privatization: towards a frictionless fitness landscape

That mobility is a crucial logic of the new fitness boom is clear in the first instance in the marketing of health and fitness apps. 'Anywhere' and 'anytime' are common refrains in the promotion of these products – understandably so, as the appeal of apps in general lies in their ease of use, especially compared to a web browser (see Anderson & Wolff, 2010), and their compatibility with mobile hardware. This was a key finding of a recent study of a small selection of prominent smartphone-compatible apps, all of which were situated in the 'health and fitness' category in online app markets (Millington, 2014). Users of MyFitnessPal, for example, an app designed for exercise and dietary tracking, are urged to partake in self-tracking anywhere and at anytime – a smartphone and a downloaded version of MyFitnessPal being all that is needed to do so. The WebMD Mobile app is promoted on the basis that trustworthy health information is available wherever one may be and whenever one should wish to seek it. In the case of MyNetDiary, also for food and exercise tracking, the consumer is mobile partly in that online support networks are themselves accessible on demand:

> MyNetDiary Community gets you the support and motivation to help you stick to your goals. . . . There is no need to drive to a meeting or weekly weigh-in since the Community and your support group are online and always available when you need them.
> (MyNetDiary Inc., 2016; cited in Millington, 2014, p. 489)

Looking more broadly, 'anywhere', 'anytime', and similar language pervades the marketing of new fitness hardware as well. The wearable device Amiigo combines wristband and shoe-clip sensors to go beyond the gym, tracking the user across all 24 hours of the day (Amiigo, 2015). Samsung's Gear Fit wrist-worn device is likewise said to be useful 24/7 (Samsung, 2016). The Basis Peak wristband – Basis being an Intel company – is portrayed as helpful 24/7 too, in its case, when it comes to heart rate tracking: "Whether working out, grabbing lunch or catching Z's, Peak tracks your heart rate all day and all night" (Basis, 2016). Fitbit offers perhaps the strongest statement along these lines in suggesting that Fitbit was built on the idea that fitness is not about gym time alone, but rather is an always-on proposition (Fitbit Inc., 2016a). Even Nintendo escaped the living room with Wii Fit U, a game that includes a wearable Fit Meter for tracking the consumer body beyond the confines of the home.

The point, all told, is that fitness technologies are designed to unburden the fitness participant from the shackles of space and time. The spirit of Charles Wesley Emerson's expressive physical culture lives on in the sense that Emerson's calisthenic system was inherently mobile, unpicked as it was from the gymnasium and the growing catalogue of exercise equipment that could be found therein. The difference, though, is that equipment is now positioned as a boon and not a burden to a mobile way of life. For Human.co, once you have downloaded the Human activity-tracking app, "The world is your gym" (Human.co, 2016).

Of course, the contrast between Emerson's view that exercise equipment hinders mobility and Human.co's view that fitness technologies enable it is not meant to suggest that mobility is newly relevant to either the fitness or technology sectors. Raymond Williams's (2004 [1974]) notion of mobile privatization is among the more famous attempts at conceptualizing the relationship between technology and space. The name 'mobile privatization' is telling. Whereas technologies could once be described as 'public technologies' – Williams gives the examples of railways and city lighting – modern industrial living in the early 1900s featured technologies that simultaneously served the causes of mobility and home-centred privatization. The automobile is the best case in point in this regard, and indeed the automobile grew more prominent at a time when industry required a great degree of mobility from the workforce, what with centralized, city-bound factory work increasingly replacing other forms of production. Yet the experience of mobile privatization did not come without consequences; as Williams (2004 [1974]) observes, it carried a need for new forms of contact. It is here that *communication* technologies become relevant. Radio helped rationalize a way of life that was ever more remote and ever more private. People could stay in touch without literally being in touch – what John Tomlinson (2007) calls 'telepresence' (also Hutchins, 2011).

Radio was thus part of the 'flood' of durable commodities entering the marketplace in the early decades of the 1900s. As Williams (2004 [1974]) writes, the trend towards mobile privatization intensified in the post-war years: "There was significantly higher investment in the privatised home, and the social and physical distances between these homes and the decisive political and productive centres of the society had become much greater" (p. 23). Television followed in radio's footsteps by rationalizing a newly intensified phase of suburbanization. As noted in Chapter 1, by the 1980s television sat alongside a number of other electronic and in many cases digital technologies in the home, including some fitness technologies. A technologically mediated household was ostensibly a self-sufficient one (Hay, 2003).

Personal computing is relevant here too, especially beginning in the 1990s with the advent of the World Wide Web. Sarah Nettleton (2004) describes the emergence of a new medical 'cosmology' at this time that she refers to as 'e-scaped' medicine. Again, the name is telling, in this case in a two-fold sense. On the one hand, through websites, newsgroups, chatrooms, and other platforms, medicine 'escaped' from formal institutions such as hospitals and clinics; said otherwise, the experience of being a patient and accessing and developing one's own medical expertise was no longer confined to these institutional sites. On the other hand, medicine is 'e-scaped' in the sense that medical knowledge and the medical body are 'informationalized' so as to 'flow' from one site to another. Taken together, the relevant point is that communication technologies helped in the process of unsettling traditional spatial dynamics. The living room or bedroom became de facto clinics in the way that treadmills made the home a de facto gymnasium. Indeed, though Nettleton's focus lies with medicine, home computing equally emboldened fitness enthusiasts, what with the capacity among fitness participants to seek out fitness information online (e.g., see Kivits, 2004).

Thus, for some time, living privately and itinerantly meant investing in the living room, other household spaces, and the car. As Dan Schiller (2007) observes, however, the recent advent of wireless forms of communication constitutes a "wrenching extension" of mobile privatization (p. 169). Mobile phones and, more recently, smartphones have come to both symbolize and facilitate a new era of connected mobility. As Stephen Groening (2010) writes with respect to television, when TV is made portable and accessible 'on demand' via mobile phones, it is not just the case that one can 'retreat' from the outside world with greater ease than ever before – though this is true. What arises is a situation whereby the notion of bringing the outside world into the living room is inverted: "the cellular phone renders the distinction between world and living room obsolete" (Groening, 2010, pp. 1339–1340). The TV-watching commuter, mobile phone in hand, is effectively 'retreating' from the outside world, but still accessing the outside world, all *while moving about the outside world* at the same time. As Groening (2010) writes, under these conditions, "the world and the living room are coterminous" (p. 1340). Human.co's claim that the world is your gym is a statement that the world and the gym share the same parameters as well.

All told, the point is that, as the fitness and technology sectors converge (see Chapter 2), fitness is impacted by a wider trend whereby technologies facilitate a more private and more mobile way of living. The new fitness boom is not just about registering and tracking one's heart rate, volumetric body fat percentage, VO2 max, and so on, but about the supposed virtues of doing so anywhere and anytime.

The question persists: what drives this wrenching extension of mobile privatization? The new fitness boom is suggestive of at least four interrelated factors.

1) Portability

This is the most obvious factor at play. In Chapter 3, we saw how contemporary fitness technologies are designed to physically connect with the body. Activity trackers are worn on the wrist, the ear, as headgear, on the torso, on the lower body, on the feet as 'shoe pods', and even internally. The point in Chapter 3 was that this allows a form of haptic monitoring – surveillance by touch – though of course what it facilitates to an equal extent is surveillance on the go.

Again, portable technologies are not entirely new. As du Gay et al. (1997) explain in recounting the story of the Sony Walkman, the cassette-playing Walkman was designed as a wearable device. In their words:

> Like the Lycra suit of the modern urban cyclist, [the Walkman] is virtually an extension of the skin. It is fitted, moulded, like so much else in modern consumer culture, to the body itself. . . . It is designed for movement – for mobility, for people who are always out and about,

for travelling light. It is part of the required equipment of the modern 'nomad' – the self-sufficient urban voyager, ready for all weathers and all circumstances and moving through the city within a self-enclosed, self-imposed bubble of sound.

(du Gay et al., 1997, pp. 23–24)

Since advertising the Walkman, Sony has moved onto other forms of wearable technology. The Sony SmartWatch 3, for example, is worn on the wrist (as the name foretells) and is promoted in part on the basis that it allows fitness tracking away from home. The promotional line, "The watch that makes life simpler and smarter" intimates a more efficient way of living (Sony Mobile Communication Inc., 2016). Yet when Sony adds that users can leave their phones behind when headed out on a run, it suggests the SmartWatch inspires mobility to an even greater extent than the communication technologies that preceded it. Elsewhere, the UA SpeedForm Gemini 2 is the company Under Armour's connected shoe. An Under Armour company blog explains that, with Gemini 2, users can leave their phones behind: "From now on, it's just you and your run" (Rahlf, n.d.). In this case, technology is made portable in the sense that it 'disappears' into other technology. The running shoe becomes a tracking technology *itself*, relieving the burden of having to carry a smartphone as exercise unfolds.

2) Fashionability

With point 1 in mind, fitness technologies – to use Sherry Turkle's (2008) language – are always on and always on you. That said, as features like heart rate tracking are made possible in transit, a question emerges as to whether fitness technologies are aesthetically appropriate for the various contexts the user might enter into and leave as part of her day. Fashionability is a second factor in the mobile privatization of fitness.

Perhaps the best case in point in this regard is the Misfit line of activity-tracking products, such as the disc-shaped Misfit Shine tracking device and its sequel product, Shine 2. Misfit was recently acquired by Fossil Group, Inc., a purveyor of wristwatches especially but also accessories like handbags. Said Fossil CEO Kosta Kartsotis in a press release announcing the Misfit purchase: "With the acquisition of Misfit, Fossil Group will be uniquely positioned to lead the convergence of style and technology and to become the fashion gateway to the high-growth wearable technology and connected device markets" (Fossil Group Inc., 2015). On Misfit's promotional website, one can find images of men and women in work attire and evening wear alongside athletes such as swimmers and skateboarders. The imagery paints a picture of refinement and athletic functionality at one and the same time.

The company iFit similarly promotes its Classic device – a stylish watch/ fitness tracker – as a resolution to the divide between fitness and fashion, and thus as appropriate for use 24 hours of the day (see iFit.com, n.d.). James Gilmore (2016) uses the neologism 'everywear' to describe the inconspicuous tethering of technologies to the body for the sake of improving physical well-being. Everywear is a play on Adam Greenfield's (2006) concept of 'everyware' – itself a play on the word *everywhere*. The idea is that, once made wearable, technology infiltrates everyday spaces, and seemingly becomes ubiquitous as a result.

Said otherwise, Gilmore attends to the corporeal dimensions of technological proliferation. Here we can add that fashionability is part of what brings contexts traditionally beyond, and perhaps even antithetical to, fitness consumerism into the purview of the new fitness boom. A business meeting is no time for a fitness assessment, unless a chic wristwatch can quietly work towards this end.

3) Functionality

Functionality goes hand-in-hand with portability as well. A sensor-enabled wristband is not just made as a bodily adornment, but is also designed to enact certain functionalities in transit – without the latter, it would surely lose its appeal.

In one sense, the combination of functionality and portability (and perhaps fashionability too) is a means for knowing the *self* in mobile fashion. The idea is that virtually any site can be made a functional site for self-improvement. Misfit provides another example here with its Speedo Shine device, a waterproof activity tracker conducive to lap counting and distance tracking in the pool (see Misfit Inc., n.d.). Even the submerged fitness enthusiast is not beyond the reaches of self-quantification. Sleep tracking is telling in this regard as well. Indeed, sleep tracking is key to the '24/7' claims made by fitness-technology merchants – '16/7' tracking or, for the restless, 17/7 or 18/7 tracking not having the same promotional ring. Simon Williams, Catherine Coveney, and Robert Meadows (2015) describe the historical trajectory of sleep tracking and analysis, focusing first on the emergence of scientific, lab-based enquiry into sleep, as realized through means such as electroencephalography (i.e., brain activity monitoring), and second on the more recent arrival at the marketplace of wearable sleep tracking technologies. A key distinction between these two forms of monitoring and analysis involves a focal shift from the 'sleep of others' to the 'sleep of ourselves'. In a time of 'm-apping' sleep – a wordplay on the concept of the mobile app – "information about sleep feeds directly back to the user, providing sleepers with new knowledge about their dormant (or not-so-dormant) body/self; knowledge that is imbued with a sense of responsibility for them to act to improve their sleep" (Williams, Coveney, & Meadows, 2015, p. 1045).

In another sense, however, knowing others, and not just oneself, is part of the remit of new fitness technologies as well, given that sharing data through bespoke and existing social media networks is a core part of the new fitness boom (see Chapter 3). Earlier, it was said how, with the app MyNetDiary, there is no need for weekly meetings since support communities are always available online. Lose It!'s vision of 'Accountability 2.0' – Lose It! being a weight-loss app described in Chapter 3 – similarly rests on the idea that an online support network lies in the palm of your hand, and is thus accessible whenever you might need it (FitNow Inc., 2016). Knowing others is a mobile pursuit.

Moreover, and in a third sense, knowing *space* in new ways is possible too. For example, the app Endomondo uses the GPS functionality of the user's smartphone to literally map out exercise routes. A recent #TrackYourArt campaign urged Endomondo users to map activity routes that double as artwork – navigating the city in the shape of a heart, for example – and to share their creations on social media. Certainly, #TrackYourArt can be read as a branding exercise (albeit one that can go south when users map out running paths in the shape of explicit images), but it is nonetheless a form of branding that exhorts the consumer towards spatial exploration and awareness.

4) Convergence

As said in Chapter 3, convergence involves compatibility across technological platforms – something that in turn allows data to flow from one platform to another (see Dwyer, 2010; Jenkins, 2006). Mobile privatization has always been contingent upon compatibility of this kind. Radio and television would have been irrelevant in the task of staying in touch while living remotely if not for broadcasting towers and, eventually, satellite technology (see Packer & Oswald, 2010).

Fitness technologies – and specifically the mobile dimensions of fitness technologies – are likewise reliant on wider, already-existing technological infrastructure. As said earlier, Endomondo's #TrackYourArt campaign is dependent upon the GPS capacities of the user's smartphone. The GPS-enabled smartphone is itself indebted to GPS satellites that serve to locate the consumer, fitness enthusiast or otherwise, in space and time. Likewise, wearable fitness trackers are reliant on the Bluetooth technology that is preloaded onto smartphones and tablets in the process of relaying fitness data from the tracking device itself to a fitness account or dashboard. Bluetooth, in other words, makes it possible to go from recording fitness data anywhere and anytime to *archiving* fitness data in much the same way. Broadband technology is important in this regard as well – for instance, mobile broadband makes fitness-related social networking possible in transit.

Furthermore, compatibility exists in that fitness technologies are generally made to work with one another, the most compelling examples of which involve compatibility across competitor devices. Google Fit, for example, is designed as a platform for storing and curating data collected across a range of health and fitness technologies, the ostensible benefit being that users can employ an array of bespoke devices – for example, an app that specializes in dietary tracking, a separate wearable device particularly adept at run tracking, and still another device made for use in the pool – without facing the need to both manage and make sense of data across multiple online platforms. Indeed, Google Fit is described as an open ecosystem made up of the following components: a fitness store where apps can both store and access data created by other apps; a sensor framework made up of representations such as data sets that make it possible to work with the data store; permissions and user controls that help establish user consent in the process of reading and storing fitness data; and Google Fit APIs (Application Programming Interfaces), which are essentially resources for creating Google Fit–supported apps on operating systems of different kinds (e.g., Android or iOS – see Google Fit, n.d.).

With Google Fit in mind, the point is that the new fitness boom is as much about constructing an ostensibly frictionless landscape for *data* as it is about exhorting consumers to think about fitness whenever they want and wherever they might be. Recall the earlier point that Sony Walkman wearers moved through the city in a self-enclosed, self-imposed bubble of sound. The bubble metaphor remains appropriate as people retreat into private experience on the go by way of their mobile devices. In the new fitness boom, however, fitness data are *spreadable* beyond the bubble (see Jenkins, Ford, & Green, 2013). We saw this in Chapter 3 – for example, with the flow of data across online networks of 'friends'. Here we can add that data potentially flow across commercial platforms of different kinds as well, including those owned and operated by different fitness merchants. In other words, mobility is both *material*, comprising the physical movement of people and their body-worn technologies, and *immaterial*, comprising the intangible movement of data through space and time. Certainly, the two are interrelated: with Google Fit, one can easily access data from a wide array of fitness technologies in the home, at the gym, and in the spaces in between.

All told, mobile privatization is wrenchingly extended indeed. As Kathleen Oswald and Jeremy Packer (2012) observe, "The media environment is no longer devoted to keeping viewers fixed on one transmission, but rather *fixed in transmission* through multiple screens that guide subjects through all of time and space" (p. 277, emphasis in original). We should not assume that, in the past, people were always stationary in communication – the car radio in particular suggests otherwise. The point is that, in keeping with John Urry's (2004) notion of 'automobility', autonomous people are urged to combine with machines made for autonomous movement as people go about their days. To use Deborah Lupton's (2012) terms, with health and fitness technologies, "the health promoter is able to insert her- or himself even more insistently into the private world of others, accessing them in any location in which their mobile device accompanies them" (p. 241). The virtual trainer can be more persistent than her human analogue ever was.

Your apps are watching you: towards an enclosed fitness landscape

And yet, we should not be so quick to announce the death of enclosure. The living room, for example, remains an important site for investment in our current era of fitness consumerism; as seen in Chapter 2, this was a core component of Nintendo's gambit in devising the Wii console in the early 2000s. Exergames and other activity-tracking devices have made their way into other institutional spaces as well, such as retirement centres, rehabilitation/ therapy contexts, and school-based PE (e.g., see Deutsch et al., 2011; Meckbach et al., 2014; Millington, 2015; Quennerstedt et al., 2013; Vander Schee & Boyles, 2010).

'Corporate wellness' is an example in this sense too. Marx (2007 [1867]) long ago made the point that capitalism requires that (blue-collar) workers reproduce themselves in order to remain productive on the factory floor. We have already seen in this book how industrialization and urbanization in the late 1800s and early 1900s were accompanied by consternation over the waning physical fitness of the workforce. Jennifer Smith Maguire (2008) makes the point that in the 1970s – the time of the first fitness boom – the private sector saw exercise as a tool for reducing health-related risks; wellness facilities and programmes were made available to (white-collar) workers as a bulwark against this.

Even more recently, Agnes Meershoek and Klasien Horstman (2016) have continued this line of critical analysis by highlighting the slew of national and international health policies (e.g., from the World Health Organization) that not only render the workplace an important site for health promotion, but ask employers to contribute to lifestyle interventions that help employees in making healthy choices in general. Private companies specializing in employee wellness have become more prominent in this context.

The *Fortune* website headline 'Fitbit Beats Back Competition with Wellness Program' bespeaks the role of fitness technologies in this latest iteration of corporate wellness (Cipriani, 2015). In the accompanying article, it is said that Fitbit has worked with thousands of companies in a corporate wellness capacity, recently announcing that employees of the retailer Target – 335,000 in number – would receive personal fitness trackers. This is effectively a side door into the fitness marketplace at a time when seemingly imposing competitors like Apple and Microsoft are likewise trying to make their way in through the front. By Fitbit's telling, the reasons for companies to invest in corporate wellness are many and include (unsurprisingly) improving employee health status and productivity. What is especially significant, however, are the means by which such outcomes can be achieved.

In Fitbit marketing, employers are told they can monitor results at both a personal and group level, with statistics on behaviour such as steps taken providing useful insight into employee performance (see Fitbit Inc., 2016b). In this sense, the features of the new fitness boom are brought to bear on employees. Corporate wellness is personalized and datafied, with Fitbit also noting that this style of wellness is fun.

Fitbit is not alone as a steward of corporate wellness. Jawbone, Lumo Bodytech, and iFit have corporate wellness offerings of their own. Garmin does too, replete with a clarion call to "Energise Your Workforce" (Garmin Ltd., 2016). Beyond its line of wearable wellness products, inclusive of wristbands, watches, and other devices, Garmin's vívohub serves as an environmental sensor for capturing data as employees adorned with Garmin wearable technologies physically pass by the sensor. One can imagine a cafeteria or break room 'kitted out' with the vívohub, the purpose being for the hub to capture data and relay them to (in Garmin's language) an overall 'wellness coordinator'. What this portends is the possibility for data, in a seemingly frictionless landscape, to flow towards a central site, and perhaps a central authority figure as well.

This idea of recentralization is key to Mark Andrejevic's (2002, 2007a, 2007b) concept of the 'digital enclosure'. Data may well 'flow' with unprecedented ease at the current moment, but data are not directionless: they flow to proprietary (enclosed) digital 'spaces', propelled in this direction in part by the fact that data are of value – literally so – in what they say about consumers. In other words, and thinking beyond corporate wellness, recentralization is a general property of our current technology landscape, and as such is an important property of the new fitness boom as well. We should not be so quick to announce the death of enclosure, understood in a material sense, nor should we overlook that enclosure, in an era of interactivity, also refers to "a variety of strategies for privatizing, controlling, and commodifying information and intellectual property" (Andrejevic, 2007b, p. 301).

Certainly, there are myriad reasons a fitness-technology company would want to compile and make use of consumer data. In Chapter 2, we saw the case of Lumo Bodytech's Data Scientist accessing 15 million consumer data points, the underlying goal being to improve the performance of Lumo technologies and enhance consumer experience in turn. Writing for Forbes, Parmy Olson (2015) describes the company Jawbone's uses (and looming uses) of consumer data as part of a social experiment whereby companies use data to engage with consumers in real time. Jawbone, for example, might 'nudge' you to watch a certain TV programme before bed based on knowledge gleaned from a range of apps that in the past you have slept well after watching that particular show. Human.co, purveyors of Human, the app that allegedly makes the world and the gym coterminous, explains that anonymized, aggregated consumer data are used to improve

Human's functionalities: "we need your data to become better at what we do" (Olmos, 2013).

But consumer data present commercial opportunities as well. Consider, for example, a study of privacy in health and fitness apps carried out by the American Federal Trade Commission (FTC) – an analysis in which it was found that the 12 apps the FTC chose to study disseminated user information to 76 third parties. As Kate Kaye (2014) explains, one app from the study sample shared information on dietary and workout habits (among other things) with 18 other entities (also see Till, 2014). Privacy Rights Clearinghouse, a California-based non-profit, came to similar conclusions in its assessment of 43 health and fitness apps, selected from both Apple and Google app markets (Ackerman, 2013). Of the study sample, 43% of free apps and 5% of paid apps shared Personally Identifiable Information (PII) with advertisers, the discrepancy explained in that paid apps by definition have an alternative revenue stream. In addition, 52% of free apps and 55% of paid apps sent out aggregated (non-PII) data to marketers. A Wall Street Journal study from the year 2010 of 101 apps from various app categories, while somewhat dated now, remains instructive for its evocative title – 'Your apps are watching you' – and for its emphasis on the economic value of consumer data. According to the report, Mobclix, an ad exchange, matches 25 ad networks with 15,000 apps seeking advertisers. In a fraction of a second, Mobclix can match app users to consumer segments defined by certain shared characteristics (Thurm & Kane, 2010).

Consumers are of course not left entirely without guidance or avenues for recourse under these conditions. Privacy policies and terms of use are ostensibly a means for ensuring informed consent in the use of health and fitness apps, including both standalone apps and those that accompany wearable technologies. If privacy policies are off-putting, in theory, there is the option to choose a competitor product, especially in a saturated app marketplace. In-app user controls are another mechanism that seemingly empower consumers. With the Apple Health app, designed in part as a data aggregator, Apple explains that consumers are ultimately in control of their own data. Consumers decide which apps can access data from the Health app, and these third party apps are required to have privacy policies of their own (Apple Inc., 2016).

Government regulation is relevant here as well as a potential bulwark against privacy breaches and, more broadly, poor practice in safeguarding consumer data. In the United States, for example, a number of laws potentially apply in the development of health-related apps, including the Health Insurance Portability and Accountability Act (HIPAA), the Federal Food, Drug, and Cosmetic Act (FD&C Act), the FTC Act, and the FTC's Health Breach Notification Rule (see Federal Trade Commission, n.d.). HIPAA, for example, is the main federal statute related to health privacy, and pertains especially to healthcare provision. In a 2015 press release, Fitbit announced that it supports

HIPAA compliance and that this would allow the corporate wellness side of Fitbit's operations to better integrate with HIPAA-covered entities (Fitbit Inc., 2016c). As Anne Marie Helm and Daniel Georgatos (2014) note, consumer protection laws (as opposed to HIPAA) have to date been most relevant when it comes to *enforcing* privacy protection. As they say of apps in general,

> To protect consumers' privacy, the FTC has pursued a number of cases against app developers whose apps surreptitiously accessed information on users' devices, typically in contravention of the apps' published privacy policies, on the legal theory that such practices are 'unfair and deceptive' under the FTC Act.
>
> (p. 160)

But there is reason to doubt that these various forms of consumer protection are in fact robust and effective enough to serve their intended cause. Start with privacy policies. In 2014, the Global Privacy Enforcement Network (GPEN) – an entity that arose in response to a recommendation by the Organisation for Economic Cooperation and Development for cross-border cooperation on privacy protection – published results of its global 'privacy sweep' of mobile apps. The sweep aimed to reproduce the consumer experience in negotiating matters such as privacy policies and data permissions with 1,211 apps of various kinds. The results, as explained by the United Kingdom's Information Commissioner's Office, were rather stark: for example, 85% of the selected apps did not clearly explain their process of collecting, using, and disclosing personal information; 59% caused difficulty for users in accessing basic privacy information; one in three appeared to request excessive permissions; and 43% did not tailor privacy communications to mobile, small-screen hardware such as smartphones (e.g., in that the typeface was too small – Information Commissioner's Office, 2014; also see Office of the Privacy Commissioner of Canada, 2014). This last point is perhaps most significant in the context of this chapter. Evidently, the marketing refrains of 'anywhere' and 'anytime' do not always apply to the matter of informed consent.

In fairness, GPEN's privacy sweep extended beyond the realm of health and fitness, considering apps from various app categories. That said, when it comes to privacy policies, the aforementioned Privacy Rights Clearinghouse study of 43 health and fitness apps is disconcerting in its own right. One major finding of this study was that 74% of free apps and 60% of paid apps had a privacy policy either in the app itself or on the developer's website, the corollary being that more than a quarter of the free apps under study and 40% of the paid apps considered in the analysis had no policy, either in-app or online (Ackerman, 2013).

Yet another study, in this case by Open Effect, a not-for-profit group affiliated with the Citizen Lab at the Munk School of Global Affairs at the

University of Toronto, offered a critical assessment of privacy policies and terms of service agreements as well (Hilts, Parsons, & Knockel, 2016). The Open Effect study is especially important due to both its recency and its focus on the hardware and software of industry-leading companies. The study sample included products from Apple, Basis (Intel), Bellabeat, Fitbit, Garmin, Jawbone, Mio, Withings, and the Chinese company Xiaomi. The research was supported by the Canadian government's Office of the Privacy Commissioner. Not unlike the Privacy Rights Clearinghouse study, Open Effect's method included both a technical analysis (e.g., that considered the security of Internet and Bluetooth transmissions) and a policy analysis – the latter leading to the conclusion that company policies threaten to reinforce, as opposed to alleviate, consumer concerns regarding the disclosure and sharing of fitness data. For example, the Open Effect research team found that companies have adopted different interpretations of personal information. Only one company (Xiaomi) explicitly stated that information collected through fitness trackers constitutes PII; in several cases, fitness data were not included in definitions of PII. In other words, personalized measures like steps taken might not, in the end, be regarded as personal information. Open Effect furthermore found it rare for companies to state in explicit terms with whom information is shared.

Two other dimensions of the Open Effect study merit consideration here as well. First, the technical aspect of the research again led to results construed by Open Effect as unsettling. For example, over a period of several months, it was found that only the Apple Watch randomized the Bluetooth Media Access Controller address it uses in Bluetooth advertising packets, leading the researchers to imagine a situation whereby a shopping centre capitalizes on this so as to pinpoint a customer's precise location and compile this with other personal information. Second, and with respect to public policy, under the auspices of an access to information provision in Canadian law, the research team issued information requests related to a research participant's use of the fitness products represented in the study. Four companies did not respond in the timeframe set out in Canadian law. The responses of the other companies varied considerably – for example, in terms of access provided to raw data.

With its technical and corporate policy findings in mind, Open Effect's recommendations for policymakers centre in part on the need to clarify precisely which data are considered personal information from a legal point of view. Indeed, in general, fitness technologies at times occupy what seems to be a liminal space in relation to public policy. For example, based on the FDA's guidance for mobile medical applications, apps that are made for individuals to "log, record, track, evaluate, or make decisions or behavioral suggestions related to developing or maintaining general fitness, health or wellness" (U.S. Food and Drug Administration, 2015, p. 25) *may* be regarded as medical devices, but are devices for which the

FDA does not intend to enforce the aforementioned FD&C Act. All told, and while Open Effect found laudable security measures in their work as well, the point is that legislation might not always be the bulwark against privacy violations that it seems on the surface, especially in a context where regulation surrounding emergent health and fitness technologies is still emerging itself.

Your apps are watching you. The phrase is instructive, as the most obvious conclusion from this analysis is that corporate *dataveillance* – originally defined by Roger Clarke (1988) as "the systematic use of personal data systems in the investigation or monitoring of the actions or communications of one or more persons" (p. 499) – is part of the 'surveillant assemblage' of the new fitness boom. That fitness technologies are designed to be always on and always on you makes sense in a context where fitness data not only serve the cause of personal optimization but also commodification. 'Old' forms of commodification have certainly not disappeared: wrist-worn trackers come at a retail cost; paid health and fitness apps have an upfront charge. In its 'new' iteration, however, commodification comprises the extraction of surplus value from fitness participation.

Indeed, a second, less obvious conclusion regarding the lasting significance of enclosure involves the blurring of labour and leisure. Information and communication technologies were already part of this trend in their ability to help extend the workday – work email being accessible without fail, for example, even away from the office (see Agger, 2011). From this perspective, corporate wellness involves leisure giving way to labour once again, as something like a leisurely walk is potentially given new meaning as a vehicle for enhancing productivity (or, perhaps, saving your employer money on insurance premiums – e.g., see Olson, 2016). At the same time, however, corporate wellness might also be construed as *leisure invading labour*, as walking – or, its datafied analogue, 'steps' – becomes an object of concern at work.

Yet even more significant is the way that fitness participation in general (i.e., and not just as part of corporate wellness programming) increasingly comprises a form of labour through what Mark Andrejevic (2002) calls the work of being watched. Media scholars have for some time pointed to the ways in which broadcasters and advertisers render consumption a site for the production of surplus value. Attention becomes a commodity when the act of watching commercials during TV broadcasts creates value beyond the cost of buying a TV set and a cable subscription. The Internet further enhanced this process, as advertising could be targeted with even greater accuracy at desired consumer demographics (see Fuchs, 2014). In the new fitness boom, running does not simply exist as a pretext for commodification – a reason to purchase Nike shoes and Under Armour shorts, for example. Instead, *running potentially becomes a commodity in its own right*, as running data are ripe for commercial exchange.

Conclusion: prosumption goes mobile

Emma Witkowski's (2015) assessment of the app Zombies, Run! (ZR) – a popular fitness app in which running regimens are taken up against the backdrop of an imagined zombie apocalypse – provides an optimistic view of the mobile nature of technologically enhanced fitness participation. Witkowski's assessment of ZR also brings together the analyses presented in Chapters 3 and 4 in many ways. ZR is, as one would expect from the name, a gamified platform: completing missions in the context of a zombie attack alleviates the tedium one might associate with running as an exercise pursuit. The game is a tracking device too, measuring the user's run as she evades the ever persistent undead. ZR also comes replete with data-sharing features, such as the option to automatically share run data on Facebook and Twitter. Based on her research into the practices and perspectives of other ZR users, as well as her own autoethnographic reflections, Witkowski (2015) makes the case that ZR furthermore allows for (re)discovery of perhaps mundane environments, inciting deeper awareness of local space. Witkowski focuses in part on the gendered significance of engaging with ZR's fictional narratives during exercise. Whereas researchers have, in the past, described the experience of embodied vulnerability when running alone (e.g., see Allen-Collinson, 2010), Witkowski argues that ZR facilitates a process whereby women reclaim risky (real) spaces as they negotiate a rather harrowing (fictional) narrative. All told, with ZR, "a socioculturally located running aesthetic (gendered, aged, economically situated and geographically placed) is being made through everyday steps into new spatial experiences and being alone, but connected, on the road" (Witkowski, 2015, p. 17).

Witkowski's account is compelling. The point of this chapter, in part, is that portability, fashionability, functionality, and convergence together have helped usher in a 24/7 fitness climate – and that this is sure to be viewed positively by many, and indeed to have many benefits.

Yet the wrenching extension of mobile privatization has inspired criticism too. For Schiller (2007), the era of wireless communication was not made to deliver playfulness and personal freedom: "It came to us, rather, as a complex historical extension of the domination and inequality that continue to define our divided societies" (p. 173). The earlier sections on openness and enclosure need be understood together. A fitness landscape in which both people and data move, seemingly without friction, is one that radically extends the parameters of data production and thus the volume and variety of data that might be expropriated for commercial purposes. In Chapter 3, the concept of prosumption was introduced to help make sense of fitness technologies and, specifically, to help conceptualize functionalities such as haptic surveillance. Here, prosumption takes on further meaning. Meershoek and Horstman (2016) make the point that health must be reified – which is to say, made knowable – if it is subsequently to be made marketable. This is precisely what prosumption-as-consumption accomplishes. We may well empower ourselves through haptic, lateral, and self-surveillance, especially as these surveillance modalities are made fun and made possible on the go. Through corporate dataveillance, the fitness landscape is also set up to empower perhaps unknown others as well.

Is this inequitable? Is it the historical extension of domination and inequality, to use Schiller's terms? Kate Crawford, Jessa Lingel, and Tero Karppi (2015) make the point that consumers have not been privy to the economic value they produce through new, interactive health and fitness technologies. The manner in which social media platforms commodify user data without sharing the profits of this commodification with consumers themselves has indeed been described as exploitative (Fuchs, 2012). At the very least, we can say that knowledge of what happens to our data is asymmetrically distributed. And the mechanisms (e.g., privacy policies) by which people might judge if they are in fact being exploited are at times quite flawed – and, moreover, that privacy protection is not always as robust as it is said to be.

In summarizing their research findings, the Open Effect team asks a series of provocative questions. Their results, they say, "Call into question the very nature of self-empowerment that is marketed alongside fitness trackers." They continue, "Can individuals be truly empowered when their data is not secured? When their data might be sold off without the individual's consent? When they cannot even learn about all the data a company has collected?" (Hilts, Parsons, & Knockel, 2016, p. 1). In a sense, the new fitness boom constitutes the realization of Charles Wesley Emerson's (1891) view that exercise should be taken up "no matter where or how [one] is situated" (p. 19) – though exercise is quantified and shared in ways that Emerson surely could not have imagined. Maybe under these conditions, we can indeed empower ourselves towards a better lifestyle, fitness technology in hand (or in shoe!). What is certain, though, is that, at the present moment, taking control of one's health and fitness in a 'responsible' way means coming to grips with a sophisticated corporate data-sharing apparatus – or, perhaps, ignoring that apparatus but then ignoring its implications as well. This is an unbalanced relationship in that companies know increasingly personal information about consumers, but data collection and sharing processes remain largely opaque to consumers themselves. Schiller's pessimism on contemporary forms of mobile privatization is indeed relevant to the new fitness boom. Your apps are watching you, and not without reason.

References

Ackerman, L. (2013). Mobile health and fitness applications and information privacy (Report to California Consumer Protection Foundation). *Privacy Right Clearinghouse*. Retrieved 27 May 2016 from www.privacyrights.org/mobile-medical-apps-privacy-consumer-report.pdf.

Agger, B. (2011). iTime: Labor and life in a smartphone era. *Time & Society*, *20*(1), 119–136.

Allen-Collinson, J. (2010). Running embodiment, power and vulnerability: Notes towards a feminist phenomenology of female running. In E. Kennedy & P. Markula (Eds.), *Women and exercise: The body, health and consumerism* (pp. 280–298). London: Routledge.

Amiigo. (2015). FAQ. Retrieved 8 July 2016 from https://amiigo.com/faq.

Anderson, C. & Wolff, M. (2010). The web is dead: Long live the internet. Retrieved 8 July 2016 from www.wired.com/magazine/2010/08/ff_webrip/.

Andrejevic, M. (2002). The work of being watched: Interactive media and the exploitation of self-disclosure. *Critical Studies in Media Communication*, *19*(2), 230–248.

Andrejevic, M. (2007a). *iSpy: Surveillance and power in the interactive era*. Lawrence: University of Kansas Press.

Andrejevic, M. (2007b). Surveillance in the digital enclosure. *The Communication Review*, *10*(4), 295–317.

Apple Inc. (2016). Privacy policy. Retrieved 8 July 2016 from www.apple.com/uk/privacy/privacy-policy/.

Basis. (2016). Retrieved 8 July 2016 from www.mybasis.com/en-GB/basis-heart-rate-monitor/.

Cipriani, J. (2015). Fitbit beats back competition with wellness program. Retrieved 8 July 2016 from http://fortune.com/2015/10/20/fitbit-wellness-program/.

Clarke, J. (1988). Information technology and dataveillance. *Communications of the ACM*, *31*(5), 498–512.

Crawford, K., Lingel, J. & Karppi, T. (2015). Our metrics, ourselves: A hundred years of self-tracking from the weight scale to the wrist wearable device. *European Journal of Cultural Studies*, *18*(4–5), 479–496.

Deutsch, J.E., Brettlera, A., Smith, C., Welsh, J., John, R., Guarrera-Bowlby, P. & Kafri, M. (2011). Nintendo Wii Sports and Wii Fit game analysis, validation, and application to stroke rehabilitation. *Topics in Stroke Rehabilitation*, *18*(6), 701–719.

du Gay, P., Hall, S., Janes, L., Mackay, H. & Negus, K. (1997). *Doing cultural studies: The story of the Sony Walkman*. Thousand Oaks: Sage.

Dwyer, T. (2010). *Media convergence*. New York: Open University Press.

Emerson, C.W. (1891). *Physical culture*. Boston: Emerson College of Oratory.

Emerson, C.W. (1900). *Expressive physical culture, or philosophy of gesture*. Boston: Emerson College of Oratory.

Federal Trade Commission. (n.d.). Mobile health apps interactive tool. Retrieved 8 July 2016 from www.ftc.gov/tips-advice/business-center/guidance/mobile-health-apps-interactive-tool#glossary.

Fitbit Inc. (2016a). Why Fitbit. Retrieved 8 July 2016 from www.fitbit.com/uk/whyfitbit.

Fitbit Inc. (2016b). Fitbit wellness. Retrieved 8 July 2016 from www.fitbit.com/uk/group-health.

Fitbit Inc. (2016c). Fitbit extends corporate wellness offering with HIPAA compliant capabilities. Retrieved 8 July 2016 from https://investor.fitbit.com/press/press-releases/press-release-details/2015/Fitbit-Extends-Corporate-Wellness-Offering-with-HIPAA-Compliant-Capabilities/default.aspx.

FitNow Inc. (2016). How it works. Retrieved 13 June 2016 from www.loseit.com/how-it-works/.

Fossil Group Inc. (2015). Fossil Group, Inc. to acquire wearable technology innovator Misfit. Retrieved 8 July 2016 from www.fossilgroup.com/investors/investor-relations/press-releases/.

Fuchs, C. (2012). The political economy of privacy on Facebook. *Television & New Media*, *13*(2), 139–159.

Fuchs, C. (2014). *Digital labour and Karl Marx*. New York: Routledge.

Garmin Ltd. (2016). Corporate wellness. Retrieved 8 July 2016 from http://sites.garmin.com/en-GB/wellness/.

Gilmore, J.N. (2016). Everywear: The quantified self and wearable fitness technologies. *New Media & Society*, *18*(11), 2524–2539.

Google Fit. (n.d.). Platform overview. Retrieved 8 July 2016 from https://developers.google.com/fit/overview.

Greenfield, A. (2006). *Everyware: The dawning age of ubiquitous computing*. Berkeley: New Riders.

Groening, S. (2010). From 'a box in the theatre of the world' to 'the world as your living room': Cellular phones, television and mobile privatization. *New Media & Society*, *12*(8), 1331–1347.

Hay, J. (2003). Unaided virtues: The (neo-)liberalization of the domestic sphere and the new architecture of community. *Television & New Media*, *1*(1), 53–73.

Helm, A.M. & Georgatos, D. (2014). Privacy and mHealth: How mobile health 'apps' fit into a privacy framework not limited to HIPAA. *Syracuse Law Review*, *64*, 131–170.

Hilts, A., Parsons, C. & Knockel, J. (2016). Every step you fake: A comparative analysis of fitness tracker privacy and security (Open Effect Report). Retrieved 8 July 2016 from https://openeffect.ca/reports/Every_Step_You_Fake.pdf.

Human.co. (2016). Retrieved 8 July 2016 from http://human.co/.

Hutchins, B. (2011). The acceleration of media sport culture. *Information, Communication & Society*, *14*(2), 237–257.

iFit.com. (n.d.). iFit® Classic. Retrieved 8 July 2016 from www.ifit.com/classic.

Information Commissioner's Office. (2014). Global survey finds 85% of mobile apps fail to provide basic privacy information. Retrieved 8 July 2016 from https://ico.org.uk/about-the-ico/news-and-events/news-and-blogs/2014/09/global-survey-finds-85-of-mobile-apps-fail-to-provide-basic-privacy-information/.

Jenkins, H. (2006). *Convergence culture: Where old and new media collide*. New York: New York University Press.

Jenkins, H., Ford, S. & Green, J. (2013). *Spreadable media: Creating value and meaning in a networked culture*. New York: New York University Press.

Kaye, K. (2014). FTC: Fitness apps can help you shred calories – and privacy. Retrieved 8 July 2016 from http://adage.com/article/privacy-and-regulation/ftc-signals-focus-health-fitness-data-privacy/293080/.

Kivits, J. (2004). Researching the 'informed patient'. *Information, Communication & Society*, *7*(4), 510–530.

Lupton, D. (2012). M-health and health promotion: The digital cyborg and surveillance society. *Social Theory & Health*, *10*(3), 229–244.

Marx, K. (2007 [1867]). *Capital: A critique of political economy, Volume 1, Part 1: The process of capitalist production*. New York: Cosimo, Inc.

Meckbach, J., Gibbs, B., Almqvist, J. & Quennerstedt, M. (2014). Wii teach movement qualities in physical education. *Sport Science Review*, 23(5–6), 241–266.

Meershoek, A. & Horstman, K. (2016). Creating a market in workplace health promotion: The performative role of public health sciences and technologies. *Critical Public Health*, 26(3), 269–280.

Millington, B. (2014). Smartphone apps and the mobile privatization of health and fitness. *Critical Studies in Media Communication*, 31(5), 479–493.

Millington, B. (2015). Exergaming in retirement centres and the integration of media and physical literacies. *Journal of Aging Studies*, 35, 160–168.

Misfit Inc. (n.d.). Speedo shine. Retrieved 8 July 2016 from http://misfit.com/products/speedo-shine.

MyNetDiary Inc. (2016). Weight loss. Retrieved 8 July 2016 from www.mynetdiary.com/whyDiary.html.

Nettleton, S. (2004). The emergence of E-scaped medicine? *Sociology*, 38(4), 661–679.

Office of the Privacy Commissioner of Canada. (2014). News release: Global privacy sweep raises concerns about mobile apps. Retrieved 8 July 2016 from www.priv.gc.ca/en/opc-news/news-and-announcements/2014/nr-c_140910/.

Olmos, R.V. (2013). Why we founded human. Retrieved 8 July 2016 from http://human.co/posts/why-we-founded-human.html.

Olson, P. (2015). A massive social experiment on you is under way, and you will love it. Retrieved 8 July 2016 from www.forbes.com/sites/parmyolson/2015/01/21/jawbone-guinea-pig-economy/#628131f2598c.

Olson, P. (2016). Fitbit's game plan for making your company healthy. Retrieved 8 July 2016 from www.forbes.com/sites/parmyolson/2016/01/08/fitbit-wearables-corporate-wellness/#6f9dd8104527.

Oswald, K. & Packer, J. (2012). Flow and mobile media: From broadcast fixity to digital fluidity. In J. Packer & S. Wiley (Eds.), *Communication matters: Materialist approaches to media, networks, and mobility* (pp. 276–287). New York: Routledge.

Packer, J. & Oswald, K.F. (2010). From windscreen to widescreen: Screening technologies and mobile communication. *The Communication Review*, 13(4), 309–339.

Quennerstedt, M., Almqvist, J., Meckbach, J. & Öhman, M. (2013). Why do Wii teach physical education in school? *Swedish Journal of Sport Research*, 1, 55–81.

Rahlf, D. (n.d.). The revolutionary smart shoe that makes you a better runner. Retrieved 8 July 2016 from https://blog.underarmour.com/devices/the-revolutionary-smart-shoe-that-makes-you-a-better-runner/.

Samsung. (2016). Gear fit. Retrieved 8 July 2016 from www.samsung.com/uk/consumer/mobile-devices/wearables/gear/SM-R3500ZKABTU.

Schiller, D. (2007). *How to think about information*. Urbana: University of Illinois Press.

Smith Maguire, J. (2008). *Fit for consumption: Sociology and the business of fitness*. New York: Routledge.

Sony Mobile Communication Inc. (2016). SmartWatch 3 SWR50. Retrieved 8 July 2016 from www.sonymobile.com/global-en/products/smartwear/smartwatch-3-swr50/#tabs.

Thurm, S. & Kane, Y.I. (2010). Your apps are watching you. Retrieved 8 July 2016 from http://online.wsj.com/article/SB10001424052748704694004576020083703574602.html.

Till, C. (2014). Exercise as labour: Quantified self and the transformation of exercise into labour. *Societies*, 4(3), 446–462.

Tomlinson, J. (2007). *The culture of speed: The coming of immediacy*. London: Sage.

Turkle, S. (2008). Always-on/always-on-you: The tethered self. In J.E. Katz (Ed.), *Handbook of mobile communication studies* (pp. 121–137). Cambridge: MIT Press.

United Nations Foundation. (2012). What we do: mHealth alliance. Retrieved 8 July 2016 from www.unfoundation.org/what-we-do/issues/global-health/mhealth-alliance.html?referrer=www.google.co.uk/.

Urry, J. (2004). The 'system' of automobility. *Theory, Culture & Society*, 21(4–5), 25–39.

U.S. Food and Drug Administration. (2015). Mobile medical applications: Guidance for industry and Food and Drug Administration staff. Retrieved 8 July 2016 from www.fda.gov/downloads/MedicalDevices/. . ./UCM263366.pdf.

Vander Schee, C.J. & Boyles, D. (2010). 'Exergaming,' corporate interests and the crisis discourse of childhood obesity. *Sport, Education and Society*, 15(2), 169–185.

Williams, R. (2004 [1974]). *Television: Technology and cultural form*. London: Routledge.

Williams, S.J., Coveney, C. & Meadows, R. (2015). 'M-apping' sleep? Trends and transformations in the digital age. *Sociology of Health & Illness*, 37(7), 1039–1054.

Witkowski, E. (2015 [Online First]). Running with zombies: Capturing new worlds through movement and visibility practices with Zombies, Run! *Games and Culture*. DOI: 10.1177/1555412015613884.

This is hard work

Negotiating technology consumption

Notebook in hand, I am sitting in a large communal space in a retirement centre in Southeastern Ontario, Canada. It's an evocative site. The walls are adorned with classic movie posters and black and white photos. An old leather golf bag with wooden clubs harkens back to an era when Arnold Palmer was as famous as Humphrey Bogart and Lauren Bacall. It's a functional space as well. The room generally serves as an activities site. Today, it has conference room-style chairs arranged in rows facing a television screen. The TV itself is mounted on a moveable stand. Jim, the retirement centre's activities coordinator, is up at the front of the room facing the TV screen, a white baton in hand. I'm sitting on the left side of the room, casually chatting with two of the retirement centre's residents who have come to partake in that day's event: Wii Bowling on the retirement centre's in-house Nintendo Wii gaming console.

This is not the first time Jim had put Wii Bowling on the activities menu at his place of work, one of four sites I visited as part of a study on exergaming in retirement centres. Nor is it strange in general to encounter a video game console in a place catering to retirees. In the years following the Wii's release, stories of retirement centres keenly adopting the Wii and, in particular, Wii Bowling, featured regularly in news media (e.g., Borland, 2007; White, 2007). As is often the case, at today's Wii session a member of staff is present to help the game move along. Jim whizzes through Wii Bowling's set-up screens – the white baton is the motion-tracking Wii Remote – and then pops into and out of the room as the activity unfolds. Another member of staff is there to help residents execute their bowling throws, launching the (virtual) ball down Wii Bowling's (virtual) alley. The game itself is a mixture of fun and frustration. Bowling throws are met with the same excitement that traditional bowling engenders. The ball's path is watched closely: there's a rising din as it approaches the pins, followed by celebration or condolences depending on the outcome. Frustration arises when the game fails to register the player's movements on screen – for example, when the on-screen avatar swings but never releases the ball, sending Wii Bowling back to a menu interface. Assistance from a member of staff is particularly useful at times such as this. At one point, after the bowler avatar yet again fails to release the on-screen ball as desired, a cry of "This is hard work!" emanates from the crowd. In the context of exergaming – emphasis on *gaming* – the commenter's wry tone was appropriate indeed (Millington, 2015).

✻ ✻ ✻ ✻ ✻

The question left lingering at this point in *Amusing Ourselves to Life* involves the matter of how people actually engage with fitness technologies – or, at least, what we know about people's experiences with fitness technologies based on research in this area to date. One way to think about consumption is to ask, 'Do fitness technologies work as they are supposed to?' 'Is my Fitbit telling me the truth when it says I took 10,000 steps today?' These are no doubt important questions. They were addressed in the introductory chapter of this book, the verdict being that fitness technologies do well at *generally* gauging fitness participation if the goal is to measure things like steps taken and energy expended. Assessing fitness technologies in this way – measuring instruments of measurement – is a matter of positivist inquiry. This chapter adopts a more constructivist paradigmatic viewpoint in examining how fitness technologies are actually put to use. Rather than asking, 'Do fitness technologies work?', the questions at hand pertain to lived experiences. What does it mean to successfully use exergaming devices? What problems might arise in such activity? What motivates people to take stock of measures of physical activity such as heart rate and calories expended? How is self-tracking actually perceived and experienced? What do people 'say' about fitness on social media? And is online dialogue about fitness in fact conducive to good health?

The theme that runs throughout this chapter is that fitness-technology consumerism is best understood as *negotiated*, which is to say that people are to some extent bound in their engagement with technologies – for example, by social norms, by their own preconceived identities, or indeed by technologies themselves – but that technology consumerism is, at the same time, far from pre-determined. People have agency. And while this is by no means a new idea, it is one that can be overlooked in research focused on fitness technologies themselves and/or their production and promotion.

The remainder of this chapter is divided into three substantive sections, followed by a conclusion. Drawing from the study described at the outset of this chapter, the first section is focused on exergaming, and considers in particular how exergames pose the challenge of synchronizing media and physical literacies – and how this challenge is dealt with in the context of retirement centres. From there, the analysis turns to the matter of self-tracking, where the negotiated nature of fitness-technology consumerism is considered as it pertains to the experience of integrating data registered through devices like fitness trackers into social life in general. Finally, section three of this chapter is focused on social media. Though platforms such as Twitter and Pinterest are not fitness technologies *per se*, they are nonetheless relevant to this analysis as sites for dialogue on fitness in general and on matters like obesity and 'fitspiration' in particular. The concluding section considers themes that cut across these foregoing sections, focusing especially on the vexed issue that fitness consumerism is evidently conducive to *both* healthy and unhealthy activity, sometimes simultaneously.

This is hard work: media and physical literacies combined

So why is exergaming hard work? The research in which Jim and others participated involved a qualitative study based in Southeastern Ontario, Canada, the rationale for the research being that while news media had covered the trend of exergaming in retirement centres in some detail, researchers had yet to respond in the same way. As noted, four retirement centres ultimately participated in the study, with data collection taking the form of interviews with retirement centre staff (mainly activities coordinators, n = 10), interviews with residents partaking in games like *Wii Bowling* and *Wii Golf* (n = 8), and participant observation of exergaming 'in action' at three of the study sites (see Millington, 2015).

A first key finding from this research was that exergaming was viewed positively by participating retirement centre staff and residents alike. This could be predicted, as the study involved members of staff who chose to use the Wii as part of their activity programming and seniors attending exergaming events, equally by choice. Even so, that exergaming was viewed as a conduit for inciting both modest physical activity benefits – even just 'getting people up' – and a sense of community in the retirement centre context is nonetheless significant. Moreover, this bespeaks a particular view of later life in general, one in which seniors, as per Nintendo marketing (see Chapter 2), are active and even avid technology users (also see Nansen et al., 2014; De Schutter, Brown, & Vanden Abeele, 2015). The activities coordinator Barb, when asked why she offered Wii gaming in the first place, responded that her motivation stemmed from the fact that seniors are her place of work are "very into" new technologies. "You saw how much fun they had," Barb said, in reference to a Wii Bowling session I had recently observed (interview, Retirement Centre C). Certainly, social class is not irrelevant here, as the participating retirement centres all catered to middle to upper class clientele. 'Active aging' in general is a discourse that directly implicates the relatively well off (e.g., see Higgs & Gilleard, 2010).

But I did indeed witness how much fun participants had when playing Wii Bowling. In this sense, it is noteworthy that Wii games were often played 'improperly'. In bowling, for instance, turns were taken at random, scores were often disregarded, and opponents cheered for one another – a communal spirit overriding a sense of competitiveness. This aligns with Denise

Copelton's (2010) finding that older persons' looked sceptically upon the use of pedometers in walking groups, given that this threatened to insert competition in place of camaraderie.

Exergaming, then, has its merits. But the second finding from this research speaks to the challenges that can arise as games like *Wii Bowling* are integrated into the retirement centre context. Injury was one concern. The participating resident Eileen described how her whole right side 'gave out' as she became a regular gamer. A member of staff at this same retirement centre spoke of seniors awakening muscles that had not been used in years. For this analysis, however, the more compelling aspect of this second finding pertains to the task of combining media and physical 'literacies'. This is where the 'hard work' of exergaming indeed rears its head.

As a concept, media literacy involves the ability "to access, analyse, evaluate and create messages across a variety of contexts" (Livingstone, 2003, p. 6; cf., Aufderheide, 1993, p. xx). As Sonia Livingstone (2003) contends, access in this regard extends beyond procurement (e.g., of hardware or software): "It must be evaluated in terms of the ongoing nature and quality of access to media technologies, contents and services" (p. 7). David Buckingham (2007) makes a similar point in noting that access involves cultural skills and competencies for using technology creatively and productively. Meanwhile, Margaret Whitehead (2001) describes physical literacy as the ability to move "with poise, economy and confidence in a wide variety of physically challenging situations" (p. 131). Whitehead's vision of physical literacy is more subjective than that proffered by others (e.g., see Tremblay & Lloyd, 2010). The point is not to measure whether movement is successful, but rather to understand physical literacy as the capacity to engage in *meaningful* activity within a wider social context.

The point that is relevant here is that the daily contexts through which we move are now technologically mediated, almost without fail. *Physical* literacy under such conditions means accessing, analyzing, evaluating, and creating content while in motion. *Media* literacy means moving with poise, economy, and confidence as one engages with technology. Let us take events unfolding at Jim's place of work as a case in point. *Wii Bowling* requires the gamer to hold a trigger button on the Wii Remote with her index finger, swing her arm in the style of a real bowling throw, and then release the trigger at the moment the on-screen avatar is set to release the virtual bowling ball. As noted, failing to enact this sequence – releasing the trigger too late, for example – brings up a menu interface that must be cleared away to have another try at the activity. For skilled gamers, such as the resident who spoke of bowling with the Wii 10 to 15 times daily, this orchestration of bodily and interpretive activity posed no problem whatsoever. But for others this proved challenging at times, prompting members of staff to intervene, whether by physically helping with the arm swing/trigger release sequencing or dealing with the menu interface so gaming could resume. Jim spoke of the frustration that can accompany ostensibly pleasurable activity:

> For people who are experiencing [the Wii] the first time, who have no experience with this type of technology, or this era of technology, they find it frustrating. You have to be standing in the right spot, you have to be pointing the right way, and sometimes people don't get that, or, you know, you've got to press button A and swing the Wii at the same time – that's challenging.
>
> (Interview, Retirement Centre D)

In relation to the Microsoft Kinect gaming system, Bjorn Nansen et al. (2014) likewise found that older persons at times had difficulty performing new, unfamiliar movements compared with younger consumers "or those who had a history of experience using different consoles" (p. 11). Jim's reference to a 'new era' of technology is telling of how even technological curiosity can be insufficient in a time of perpetual technological innovation (see Chapter 2). The general point here is that, while combining media and physical literacies might well be straightforward for some, and while the technologies of times' past certainly implicated the body, the lived experience of the new fitness boom means synchronizing interpretive and movement capacities on a new and even more challenging scale.

Finally, the third finding from this research was that members of care staff likewise face challenges in integrating new technologies into the retirement centre context. Media and physical literacies are required on their part too, given their role in setting up exergame events, teaching residents how to play, and, as seen earlier, intervening as necessary. While thus far in *Amusing Ourselves to Life* we have seen how various forms of expertise are relevant to the new fitness boom – that of engineers, of data scientists, of (human) health and fitness experts, and of technologies-cum-anthropomorphic coaches and trainers, among others – the support of care staff in, for example, intervening in Wii gaming is reflective of Maria Bakardjieva's (2005) concept of the 'warm expert': the person who "mediates between the technological universal and the concrete situation, needs and background of the novice user with whom he [sic] is in a close personal relationship" (p. 99). On the matter of gaming among older persons in domestic contexts, Bob De Schutter, Julie Brown, and Vero Vanden Abeele (2015) likewise describe how some respondents in their research were introduced to digital games by others, in turn developing "new game-based relationships in order to learn about and eventually master the new technology" (p. 5). Exergaming, and, in general, fitness-technology consumerism, might indeed be hard work. The point of warm expertise is to alleviate this.

Thus, the findings from this research suggest a form of constrained agency as older persons negotiate Wii hardware and software with various ends in mind – sociality, fitness, and fun most notable among them. It would seem at first glance that these findings are of relatively narrow significance, pertaining as they do to institutional sites catering to retirees. Thinking on a slightly broader level, however, we should expect that exergaming in other contexts will likewise involve a degree of latitude from gamers – though not complete freedom – as they engage with the structure that particular games provide. In researching exergaming in school-based PE, for example, Jane Meckbach et al. (2014) found that games of different kinds inspire both different types of movement and different forms of interactivity. In Wii Fit Plus, young people interacted only with the gaming interface, whereas sport and dance games led participants to engage with one another as well.

On an even broader scale, the notion of combining literacies of different types has purchase in thinking about technology consumerism in general. It is reasonable to expect that playing Wii Fit, checking one's progress on a smartwatch mid-exercise, or mapping one's route on a fitness app all require the deft synchronization of media and physical literacies, much as Wii Bowling evidently does – though, certainly, this is a matter requiring further empirical attention. Fitness technologies have to date been construed as 'biopedagogical' devices: 'bio', as in Foucault's notion of biopower, whereby power-effects are exerted over and through the body, and pedagogy, in the sense that teaching and learning take place beyond the classroom walls (see Fotopoulou & O'Riordan, 2017; Wright & Harwood, 2009). Given the sophisticated functionalities of devices like wearable fitness trackers, people are certainly bound to learn in variegated ways in their use of fitness technologies. Self-tracking, for example, might teach someone about his or her performance in a certain activity over time (as explored next). But what Wii Bowling demonstrates, even in its simplicity – or perhaps because of it – is the fundamental idea that technology consumerism both requires and provides grounds for developing poise, economy, and confidence of movement *and* the ability to access, analyse, evaluate, and/or create content. More to the point, interpretative and embodied capacities are *brought together*: they must be enacted simultaneously for pleasurable experience not to be arduous in the end. To stay with the teaching and learning theme, biopedagogies require literacies of different kinds.

Quantifying the self: the lived politics of self-tracking

Self-tracking, as said earlier, is the second issue to consider in this analysis. As seen in previous chapters, this is perhaps the most celebrated dimension of the new fitness boom. What does the literature tell us about the lived experiences of those partaking in such activity?

The Quantified Self (QS) community, or movement, as it is sometimes understood (see Choe et al., 2014), is a good starting point for answering this question. QS got its start in 2007 when *Wired* magazine editors Gary

Wolf and Kevin Kelly started a blog called quantifiedself.com, a site for 'QSers' to share information on the practice of measuring – often in intimate and meticulous detail – various aspects of the body and daily life. Based on a study of QS-themed *Wired* articles from the years 2008 to 2012, Minna Ruckenstein and Mika Pantzar (2017) argue that four themes permeate *Wired*'s vision of self-quantification:

- Transparency, which is to say the free and open sharing of data on topics related to exercise, sexual activity, bowel movements, and far beyond.
- Optimizing, a theme that bespeaks the possibility of living – through data – "better, faster, and stronger" (Ruckenstein & Pantzar, 2017, p. 408).
- Feedback loops, meaning that data, when presented in a digestible and actionable way, can inform behaviour and, if necessary, behaviour change.
- And, finally, 'biohacking' – the idea that QSers are inclined to creatively and eagerly experiment with virtually all aspects of their lives.

All told, these four themes converge to form a 'dataistic' paradigm (Van Dijck, 2014) whereby data are granted a powerful and even agentic role. Data both reveal and *suggest* ways of being.

Against the backdrop of *Wired*'s dataism, the structure of QS community meet-ups provides a window onto actual QS experiences, given that these meet-ups tend to follow a show and tell-style format consisting of three questions: What did you do? How did you do it? What did you learn? Choe et al. (2014) examined 52 QSer videos addressing these questions, posted between the years 2008 and 2013. On the matter of 'what they do', Choe et al. found that activity (40% of QSers), food (31%), weight (29%), sleep (25%), and mood (13%) were most commonly tracked. Other tracked items related mainly, though not exclusively, to health and fitness, such as cognitive performance, blood glucose, heart rate, stress, body fat, and posture. On the 'how' question, commercial hardware such as Fitbit trackers and heart rate monitors were most commonly used for data collection (56% of QSers). The 'what did you learn question' is perhaps most compelling. Choe et al. describe how QSers are often led via descriptive statistics and correlations to *qualitative* take-away points – in one case, for example, the view that small things in life are the main contributors to one's happiness.

This last point is telling. As Gavin Smith and Ben Vonthethoff (2017) contend based on their own examination of QSer videos (numbering 30 in their case), for QS participants, quantification appears to inspire a process of 'becoming with' data. That is to say, while data can certainly serve as an external force, 'speaking for' the bodily referents from which they are derived, a kind of reciprocal engagement also emerges whereby the self-tracker is involved in generating and defining data, "as much as the data objectivates and subjectivates the body/self" (Smith & Vonthethoff, 2017,

p. 17). To give a concrete case in point, Smith and Vonthethoff describe one QS participant who initially contested his heart rate monitor's feedback loop, but eventually came to accept it – human intuition and machine-based insights spiralling together and, for a time, finding themselves at loggerheads. Dawn Nafus and Jamie Sherman (2014) go a step further in this regard in arguing that QSers engage in what they label 'soft resistance'. Again, Nafus and Sherman (2014) recognize that, for QSers like participant Michael, who eagerly self-quantifies with the help of various technologies, data can indeed act in an objectifying way. Yet soft resistance arises as identity categories – so crucial to industry in mapping consumer archetypes through data – are acknowledged, and perhaps even 'used', but only as a kind of starting point in understanding the self. QSers privilege idiosyncrasy – the 'n' of one is what matters – and thus can (softly) resist the notion of working towards generalized and pre-ordained ideals, including in the realms of health and fitness.

The question remains, however: what does self-tracking mean for those not explicitly defining themselves as self-quantifiers? We can begin to answer this question through survey research that has unearthed self-tracking trends in a big picture sense. With a sample of 3,014 American adults, the U.S.-based Pew Research Center's Tracking for Health survey is often cited for these purposes (Fox & Duggan, 2013). Arguably, the most eye-catching finding from this study is that 69% of respondents track some kind of health indicator for themselves or someone else, with 60% tracking weight, diet, or exercise. 'Drilling down' into these data, Eulàlia Puig Abril (2016) focused more specifically on those who made up this 60% figure – 530 respondents in all. On the one hand, Abril's (2016) contribution is to highlight demographic trends in weight, diet, and exercise tracking, the main take-away point being that "those who self-tracked [weight, diet, and exercise] were females with a higher socioeconomic status who used the Internet and mobile technologies more than those not self-tracking" (p. 6). This is a picture of relative privilege. On the other hand, Abril notes that using a mobile device was related to a higher tracking frequency and better overall (self-judged) health status, even though only 9% of the sample in question in fact utilized a mobile technology for such purposes. It need be remembered here that the Pew survey data was collected in 2012 – long ago on the timescale of technological change – meaning this 9% figure is likely now to be low.

Indeed, in work published three years later, Paul Krebs and Dustin Duncan (2015) found that more than 58% of the 1,604 mobile phone users they surveyed had downloaded a health-related mobile app, with fitness and nutrition apps registering as most commonly used. A total of 58.4% of respondents had used 1–5 health apps; 13.4% had used more than 20! Krebs and Duncan (2015) compare their own results to the Pew survey. "Similar to our findings," they write, "the Pew survey indicated that younger persons and those with higher incomes and education were more likely to use a health app" (p. 8), though gender was not a factor for Krebs and Duncan (2015) in the same way it was in the Pew survey. These findings reflect the company Nielsen's results, elicited through a general population survey of 3,956 adults aged 18 or over, that fitness band owners tend to be young and tend to have more income at their disposal than non-owners (The Nielsen Company, 2016). Krebs and Duncan (2015) furthermore note that respondents deemed 'obese' by way of BMI were 11% more likely to use a health app than those falling in the 'normal' range. Most respondents in their research felt that health apps had improved their health, though 45.7% of respondents had stopped using some apps due to reasons of 'data entry burden' (e.g., the need to manually input data), loss of interest, or hidden costs. This latter point reflects the statistic that one-third of Americans stop using their wearable device within six months of acquiring it (Arthur, 2014).

The flip side of disengagement is of course motivation. H. Erin Lee and Jaehee Cho (2016) investigated the latter, using a survey of 142 university students to examine intentions to continue using diet and fitness apps. Lee and Cho were unsurprised to find that 'recordability', 'networkability', credibility, comprehensibility, and trendiness all emerged as important factors in sustaining app consumerism – the first of these being especially important in the context of this discussion, given that 'recordability' is crucial to self-tracking over time. By contrast, accuracy and entertainment were *not* found to be significant predictors of intentions to continue app use among survey respondents. For Lee and Cho, this was surprising and, in the case of entertainment, deemed out of step with previous research on why people select and use many forms of communication technology (e.g., Ferguson & Perse, 2000).

At the same time, qualitative research provides more textured insight into lived experiences of self-tracking and, more broadly, technology consumerism. John Rooksby et al. (2014) carried out research with 22 participants employing a range of technologies for self-tracking purposes, including physical devices like wrist-worn trackers, exergames, and apps. Five styles of personal tracking emerged out of this work:

- Directive tracking, meaning self-tracking towards a particular goal, such as walking 10,000 steps a day.
- Documentary tracking, aimed at (as the name suggests) documenting activity as opposed to changing it – for example, knowing how many steps it takes to get to work.
- Diagnostic tracking, which is to say, tracking aimed at solving a problem like fatigue, and can therefore have an 'expiry' date once a solution is determined.
- Collecting rewards, including material rewards – two participants were using an app that transferred small payments from those failing to meet their activity goals to those succeeding in doing so.

- And, finally, fetishized tracking, meaning data collection simply for the sake of it.

Beyond this typology, Rooksby et al. (2014) note that personal tracking has a certain sociality to it. In one sense, they describe tracking as a 'co-present' activity, meaning something done among families, friends, and co-workers. Elsewhere, for example, Jennifer Whitson (2015) highlights the case of 4-year-old Luka and his dad – both Fitbit wearers – who invented and partook in real-life games as a way of upping their daily step count, with the promise of Fitbit accomplishment badges pending as a reward (see Chapter 4). Tracking is both a personal and social experience.

In another, related sense, Rooksby et al. (2014) describe self-tracking as part of the 'felt life', meaning it is often indissociable from highly personal matters such as one's sense of self-esteem. Paula Gardner and Barbara Jenkins (2016) pick up on a similar theme, in their case through an experimental methodological approach that had participants engage with electroencephalogram (EEG, for monitoring the brain) and electrocardiogram (ECG, for monitoring the heart) technologies and the data they produce. It is worth noting for these purposes that heart rate tracking via ECG is now a functionality of commercial fitness technologies such as smart clothing. As seen in Smith and Vonthethoff's (2017) and Barta and Neff's (2016) research on the QS, for Gardner and Jenkins's (2016) participants, data in one sense yielded a sense of alienation – the self was suddenly made strange. Yet participants also worked past this experience and its attendant frustrations. ECG and EEG readouts were playfully manipulated. Graphical visualizations of data were reinterpreted through other dimensions of life, such as familiar landscapes, soundscapes, and buildings. Gardner and Jenkins (2016) describe this as 'affective labour', pertaining as it does to the notion that data are *felt*. In this sense, the process of 'datafying' one's self is affected by one's preconceived experiences and sense of identity. As Gardner and Jenkins (2016) say, participants "'tarried' with memory, experience, and pleasurable forms of embodiment to create more complex narratives in the virtual spaces between the linear points of their digital biodata representations" (p. 5).

All told, the empirical literature on self-tracking reads as an implicit, and at times explicit, rejoinder to scholarly critiques of health and fitness technologies – including critiques levied thus far in this book! That consumers often find benefits in using devices like health and fitness apps cannot be overlooked. Even the fact that technologies are commonly discarded after a short stint does not mean they were altogether useless; they may simply have served their purpose. Moreover, whereas Ruckenstein and Pantzar (2017) critique *Wired*'s dataistic paradigm for obscuring the politics of knowledge production (i.e., by obscuring the processes and practices through which data are made meaningful), empirical accounts construe data production as dialogical and subjective. Data are negotiated as part of QSers' wider experiences, and it would seem that, in general, self-trackers understand their 'data doubles' in a similar way (see Ruckenstein, 2014). Many health promoters would surely be encouraged by Krebs and Duncan's (2015) finding that those with an elevated BMI are more likely to be drawn to mobile health and fitness apps.

Yet we should also be reluctant to uncritically praise fitness technologies in light of what we know from research on the lived dimensions of self-tracking. As survey studies have shown – and as we should expect – technology consumerism generally favours those with the spending power to consume. Two other, related points should equally temper our optimism.

In one sense, the sociality of self-tracking means such activity is affected by social life in *all* its complexities. Consider, as an example here, Nanna Gorm and Irina Shklovski's (2016) study of a three-week, work-based step-counting programme where employees used a range of tracking devices in pursuing a goal of 10,000 steps per participant per day. Non-participants declined to engage in this programme for several reasons, such as concerns over the blurring of boundaries between labour and leisure. Of equal interest is the finding that even those partaking in the step-count initiative soon found how revealing data disclosure could be, with the step count measure acting as a platform for workplace dialogue on what people do (or do not do) outside of work. As another example here, Jessica Francombe-Webb (2016) studied 12- and 13-year-old girls' uses of the cheerleading (and calorie counting) exergame *We Cheer* (also see Francombe, 2010). Francombe-Webb (2016) found that, while the game's idealized depictions of thinness and hyper-femininity were in one sense viewed as unrealistic, in contradictory fashion they were also reaffirmed. The latter was true both in that 'flabby' bodies were decried and in that participants at times expressed a desire to achieve the thin bodies they saw on screen. In other words, the experience of consuming *We Cheer* takes place in a social context where the body is always-already value laden (also see Depper & Howe, 2017).

In a second, related sense, the idea that people bring their own pre-formed experiences and identities to bear on the process of generating and interpreting data – tarrying with memory, for example – might not necessarily make technology consumerism more rewarding. Hayeon Song, Wei Peng, and Kwan Min Lee (2011) investigated how people with relatively high or low self-esteem engaged with *EyeToy: Kinect*, an exergame that allows gamers to see their actual self on screen beside a virtual trainer. While a positive effect might be expected for all participants in this research, the game, in this case, was found to have a *negative* impact on people of high body image dissatisfaction, as the 'imperfect' self was contrasted with the (virtual) ideal standard. Whether datafied *representations* of the body have the same effect is unclear, though many of the aforementioned studies indeed highlight how data are often felt to be objectifying in the first instance. The prospect of 'becoming with' data, to use Smith and Vonthethoff's (2017) phrase, does not render this objectifying experience completely irrelevant.

Jordan Etkin's (2016) research on the unintended consequences of personal quantification is relevant here as well. Through six experiments, two of which focused on physical activity, Etkin found that while measurement generally increases activity output (e.g., steps taken), it simultaneously tends to *decrease* the enjoyment people derive from the activity in question. Measurement has a certain seductiveness to it, Etkin (2016) argues, but what it also tends to do is replace intrinsic with extrinsic motivation. The latter makes activities like walking seem more like work, and in general extrinsic motivation is deemed much less effective than intrinsic motivation in sustaining engagement. By Etkin's account, measurement has hidden costs.

Feeling fitspired? Fitness and social media

The third and final element to consider in this chapter pertains to online experience, and specifically the role of social media in contemporary fitness cultures. Twitter, Facebook, Instagram, Pinterest, and other platforms provide opportunities for fitness enthusiasts to network and share information in lateral fashion. Moreover, and as seen in earlier chapters, fitness consumers are oftentimes 'pushed' in these directions by fitness merchants (e.g., through the option to automatically share workout results on Twitter) and are equally encouraged to use the networking features that are unique to particular products and services (e.g., an app-hosted online community). Social media in general has been celebrated for its capacity to put consumers themselves at the forefront of content creation: tweets are ostensibly unfiltered. While this is debatable – automatically uploaded tweets have been filtered through a particular fitness technology, for example – exploring the intersections of fitness and social media to some extent unearths a view from below, or from fitness participants themselves.

In the first instance, scholarly literature is helpful in delivering general insight into what happens when people communicate about fitness online. Theodore Vickey, Kathleen Martin Ginis, and Maciej Dabrowski (2013) offer initial guidance on this matter through their study of nearly 2 million English-language tweets linked to hashtags for five prominent mobile fitness apps: Endomondo, MyFitnessPal, Nike+, RunKeeper, and dailymile. From this exceedingly large pool of data, these researchers in turn adopted a grounded approach in devising a typology of content, one that divided tweets into three categories: 'Activity' tweets (73% of the study sample) listing either workout results on their own or with some additional information (e.g., on the weather or how one felt, post-exercise); 'Conversation' tweets (21%), further subdivided by the researchers into tweets pertaining to technical support, corporate marketing (e.g., press releases), statements of support from other tweeters, and the sharing of fitness information; and finally

'Blarney' (5%), further classified as either pointless babble or spam. What stands out, at least in part, to Vickey, Ginis, and Dabrowski (2013) from these results is the lack of meaningful and engaged conversation between fitness enthusiasts on Twitter. Only about a fifth of the sampled tweets were devoted to conversation, and a small portion of these went towards technical issues and marketing. Twitter, then, is being used quite readily, but it would seem it is being used "more as a one-way, one-to-many publishing service than a two-way, peer-to-peer communication network" (Vickey, Ginis, & Dabrowski, 2013, p. 311).

Of course, this should not be taken to mean that reciprocal and profound forms of social networking never take place online. As noted earlier with respect to Lee and Cho's (2016) study of diet and fitness apps, 'network-ability' was found to be an important factor in intention to continue using such products. Urban Carlén and Ninitha Maivorsdotter (2017) examined online engagement on a social networking site made specifically for runners, highlighting that online exchanges – for instance, in relation to technology-generated workout results – indeed took place and tended to be quite positive. Conversations sometimes involved running invitations, suggesting that dialogue can move offline, having started through networking services. As seen in Chapter 3, many technology merchants also take the step of gamifying social networking as a way of propelling interactivity. The online service Fitocracy, which includes features such as inter-user 'duels', was highlighted in Chapter 3 as one case in point. In surveying 200 Fitocracy users, Hamari and Koivisto (2015a) found that social factors such as the perception of reciprocal benefit relate positively among those on Fitocracy to the experience of using the service and to exercise continuance – as well as to respondents' intention to recommend Fitocracy to others (also see Hamari & Koivisto, 2015b). On the whole, between mainstream and bespoke platforms, fitness enthusiasts have a range of mechanisms for engaging with one another, and for engaging in both profound and 'shallow' ways.

Another way to assess what fitness 'looks like' on social media is to consider how *specific* issues are discussed on Twitter and its social media kin. Weight discourse is relevant in this regard, given that overweight and obesity are generally understood as antithetical to fit living. In this vein, Jiyeon So et al. (2015) focused their social media analysis on the 30 most retweeted tweets related to each of four keywords – obese, obesity, overweight, and fat – over a two-month time period in 2012. What So et al. (2015) found in the first instance is that retweets tend to be evocative and humorous. Amusing tweets, for example, had a retweet frequency of 78.8%; by contrast, 'anger' retweets registered a score of just 3.7%. Looking deeper into these data, 60.64% of humorous retweets involved derogatory jokes – something that, for So et al. (2015), "provides yet another piece of empirical evidence demonstrating the omnipresence of weight stigma in social media" (p. 11). Janet Lydecker et al. (2016) arrived at a similar conclusion in examining more than 4,500 tweets containing the word 'fat', as collected over a four hour period in 2013. In this sample, 56.6% of messages were coded as negative, 32.1% were deemed neutral, and just 9.9% were found to be positive – a set of findings that led Lydecker et al. (2016) to conclude that weight stigmatization is present on Twitter, much as it is offline as well.

Of course, we should not overlook that 'anger' retweets in So and colleagues (2015) research included anger over stigmatization and that nearly 40% of humorous retweets involved non-derogatory jokes. These findings can be set alongside Courtney Szto and Sarah Gray's (2015) finding that 97 of the 524 tweets they analyzed as part of their research into Twitter discourse on the weight loss–themed TV programme *The Biggest Loser* resisted the show's rather straightforward and functionalist narratives on losing weight. People questioned, for example, the idea that eating healthily on a budget was as easy as the show suggests. Even so, Szto and Gray (2015) arrive at the familiar conclusion that Twitter discourse does more to perpetuate prevailing (and, in their view, problematic) obesity rhetoric than contest it.

Another way of examining specific fitness-related issues on social media is to look at the term 'fitspiration' – now popular in the process of sharing user-generated fitness content. Courtney Simpson and Suzanne Mazzeo (2017) offer insight into what fitspiration content comprises through their study of 1,050 Pinterest posts, or 'pins', selected via the keyword 'fitspiration' and its derivatives, 'fitsporation' and 'fitspo'. Evidently, fitspiration is a decidedly gendered construct, at least in Simpson and Mazzeo's study sample. Of the sampled posts that included an image of a person (85% of the total sample), 97.2% of people depicted were women; 67.9% were white. Just as important is what these posts promoted. As Simpson and Mazzeo (2017) write, "The majority of fitspiration content promoted weight management standards and behaviors as a way to be thin, fit, sexy, or beautiful" (p. 564). In other words, fitspiration appears more connected to body image than to health.

Fitspiration in this regard is not far off from 'thinspiration' – a term that, when searched on Pinterest, elicits a warning message about disorderly eating (Lewallen & Behm-Morawitz, 2016). In contrasting fitspiration and thinspiration websites, Leah Boepple and Kevin Thompson (2015) found they both "contained thematic content about women's body weight, thinness, weight, and eating guilt, restriction, stigmatization, and objectification" (p. 100) – though thinspiration sites generally did contain more content of this kind. In this sense, it is perhaps unsurprising that researchers have found cause for concern in people's actual engagement with fitspiration content. Reporting results from their research with 118 women, Lewallen and Behm-Morawitz (2016) note that the amount of fitness 'pinboards' followed by participants on Pinterest predicted intentions to engage in extreme weight-loss tactics – fad dieting, for example. Marika Tiggemann and Mia

Zaccardo (2015) arrived at similar findings in their research, carried out with 130 female undergraduates, on fitspiration and Instagram. As Tiggemann and Zaccardo (2015) write based on their results: "exposure to fitspiration images resulted in greater body dissatisfaction and lower state appearance self-esteem than did exposure to control (travel) images" (p. 65). Adding to this concern is the fact that, in the context of social media, hashtags such as #fitspiration and #thinspiration can be partnered with broader terms such as #fitness in order to bring fitspo and thinspo content to a wider pool of consumers than it otherwise might reach (Ghaznavi & Taylor, 2015).

It is worth noting as well that Tiggemann and Zaccardo (2015) found that fitspiration fulfilled its ostensible purpose. Fitspiration *fitspired*: upon seeing fitspo images, participants were motivated to both eat healthily and improve their level of fitness. While in broad terms, this section shows that social media serve a range of purposes – from declarative tweets on workout results to gamified social networking to engagement around specific topics such as #fitspiration – in Tiggemann and Zaccardo's (2015) work we also arrive back at a familiar problem. Just as Etkin (2016) found that measurement increases output but decreases intrinsic motivation, fitspiration can evidently live up to its name while also having far less desirable effects.

Conclusion: active audiences, rational actors

In assessing the Quantified Self movement, Dawn Nafus and Jamie Sherman (2014) conclude by suggesting that QSers do not escape the understanding of healthiness embedded in devices such as wrist-worn fitness trackers so much as a wrestle with dominant notions of what healthiness entails. This is soft resistance at work. Data may well have agency in their own right – for example, in suggesting where daily life is going right and wrong – but people are far from "mindless dupes" in making sense of what data mean (Nafus & Sherman, 2014, p. 1793).

This insight from Nafus and Sherman's (2014) work is instructive in a twofold sense. The language of mindless dupes – whether Nafus and Sherman's intention or not – reflects the view in the tradition of media audience research that people are not necessarily swayed by what they see on TV or in media of other kinds. The audience construct itself has not aged well over time. Audiences have for some time been understood as institutional fictions (e.g., of media industries – Hartley, 1992; also see Alasuutari, 1999; Millington & Wilson, 2010). The notion of clearly delineated and easily identifiable audiences has only become more specious as people have taken a more active role in developing media texts of their own. Nonetheless, the presumption at the heart of Stuart Hall's (1993) landmark commentary on media encoding/decoding remains relevant still: people have agency, even if their agency is constrained by factors such as their personal backgrounds or how the media text in question is encoded in production in the first place. Indeed, this fundamental idea is borne out in the preceding analysis. Exergamers work within a gaming structure and evidently must develop certain literacies to make games like *Wii Bowling* worthwhile. At the same time, though, they might evade certain elements of the gaming structure in the interest of (for example) camaraderie and fun. So too might they receive assistance from warm experts in using gaming hardware and making sense of gaming software. In a similar vein, self-tracking is evidently a negotiated experience, and not just for QSers. An ECG readout might be alienating in the first instance, but people can also tarry with data so that data make sense vis-à-vis their sense of identity and/or in the context of social life in general. Social media, for their part, elicit a range of opportunities for creating and sharing knowledge about fitness experience. At their most compelling, platforms such as Twitter allow fitness devotees to contest prevailing notions of what fit and unfit living comprise. As best we can tell from empirical research, fitness-technology consumers are not mindless dupes, but rather are active and at times critical in using the devices and platforms examined in this book.

At the same time, Nafus and Sherman's (2014) reference to wrestling with *healthiness* in particular is of course relevant to this discussion. A theme running throughout this book is the salience of healthism (and existing critiques of healthism) to the new fitness boom – healthism being an ideology whereby health is deemed predominantly a matter of personal responsibility (Crawford, 1980, 2006). Negotiated consumerism might well be viewed by some as the province of the rational health actor. People not only have a range of (consumer) health and fitness options at their disposal at the current moment in time, but, if the earlier conclusions about negotiated consumerism are accepted, so too do they have the capacity to wrestle with these options, accepting the ones they like and discarding those found unhelpful. The finding from Krebs and Duncan's (2015) research that some smartphone owners download upwards of 20 health and fitness apps, parsing good from bad, would likely be read by some as a vindication of the neoliberal health imperative. At the very least, it presents critical scholars with an intriguing question: if people are not mindless dupes, why not trust personal empowerment as the primary health promotion mechanism?

Healthism can be critiqued along numerous lines, many of which have been taken up already in this book. With the analysis presented in this particular chapter in mind, however, a first problem emerges in that the responsibility mantra overlooks the very obvious barriers to partaking in health consumerism in the first place. Fitness technologies have been found to be tools for the relatively privileged: access in the first instance is contingent on spending power, as Krebs and Duncan (2015) also suggest. Understood broadly, access can evidently be complicated by the need for literacies in the right combination as well.

More to the point, a key problem with conflating *negotiated* fitness consumerism and rational/responsible health activity is that it overlooks the many complexities that characterize – or, we might say, bedevil – the pursuit of healthy, 'empowered' living. Indeed, the earlier sections on self-tracking and social media in particular reveal a rather vexing issue: that ostensibly healthy activity can work to quite the opposite effect. In self-tracking, for example, and as Etkin (2016) contends, measurement might increase output, as determined through a metric like steps taken, yet it can simultaneously make walking feel like work as it trades intrinsic for extrinsic motivation. Moreover, tracking oneself on screen can evidently be detrimental to those utilizing an exergame like *EyeToy Kinect* with a sense of bodily dissatisfaction already in place. With social media, fitspiration has been shown to fitspire, but it has also been shown to be something that can heighten bodily dissatisfaction in the process. This is in addition to the fact that people might well encounter weight stigma as they go online to seek out information – or, indeed, to be inspired.

No doubt, it is true that responsibility plays a part in living healthily. Moreover, it is worth remembering that many uses of fitness technologies seem rather mundane and functional, as outlined earlier. The point is that, while the selling of fitness technologies generally pivots around the idea of responsibility, filtered through terms such as 'empowerment' and 'optimization', responsible, healthy living is generally an option for the relatively privileged to begin with, and is not so simple and straightforward even among those with the capacity to consume. The complexities of fitness consumerism reveal fault lines in the health responsibility mantra.

References

Abril, E.P. (2016). Tracking myself: Assessing the contribution of mobile technologies for self-trackers of weight, diet, or exercise. *Journal of Health Communication*, 21(6), 638–646.

Alasuutari, P. (Ed.). (1999). *Rethinking the media audience: The new agenda*. Thousand Oaks: Sage.

Arthur, C. (2014). Wearables: One-third of consumers abandoning devices. Retrieved 17 August 2016 from www.theguardian.com/technology/2014/apr/01/wearables-consumers-abandoning-devices-galaxy-gear.

Aufderheide, P. (Ed.). (1993). *Media literacy: A report of the national leadership conference on media literacy*. Aspen: Aspen Institute.

Bakardjieva, M. (2005). *Internet society: The internet in everyday life*. London: Sage.

Barta, K. & Neff, G. (2016). Technologies for sharing: Lessons from quantified self about the political economy of platforms. *Information, Communication & Society*, 19(4), 518–531.

Boepple, L. & Thompson, J.K. (2015). A content analytic comparison of fitspiration and thinspiration websites. *International Journal of Eating Disorders*, 49(1), 98–101.

Borland, S. (2007). Elderly 'addicted' to Nintendo Wii at care home. Retrieved 18 August 2016 from www.telegraph.co.uk/news/uknews/1563076/Elderly-addicted-to-Nintendo-Wii-at-care-home.html.

Buckingham, D. (2007). *Media education: Literacy, learning and contemporary culture*. Cambridge: Polity Press.

Carlén, U. & Maivorsdotter, N. (2017). Exploring the role of digital tools in running: The meaning-making of user-generated data in a social networking site. *Qualitative Research in Sport, Exercise and Health*, 9(1), 18–32.

Choe, E.Y., Lee, N.B., Lee, B., Pratt, W. & Kientz, J.A. (2014). Understanding quantified-selfers' practices in collecting and exploring personal data. *CHI '14, Proceedings of the SIGCHI Conference on Human Factors in Computing Systems*, 1143–1152.

Copelton, D.A. (2010). Output that counts: Pedometers, sociability & the contested terrain of older adult fitness walking. *Sociology of Health & Illness*, 32(2), 304–318.

Crawford, R. (1980). Healthism and the medicalization of everyday life. *International Journal of Health Services*, 10(3), 365–388.

Crawford, R. (2006). Health as a meaningful social practice. *Health*, 10(4), 401–420.

Depper, A. & Howe, P.D. (2017). Are we fit yet? English adolescent girls' experiences of health and fitness apps. *Health Sociology Review*, 26(1), 98–112.

De Schutter, B., Brown, J.A. & Vanden Abeele, V. (2015). The domestication of digital games in the lives of older adults. *New Media & Society*, 17(7), 1170–1186.

Etkin, J. (2016). The hidden cost of personal quantification. *Journal of Consumer Research*, 42(6), 967–984.

Ferguson, D.A. & Perse, E.M. (2000). The World Wide Web as a functional alternative to television. *Journal of Broadcasting & Electronic Media*, 44(2), 155–174.

Fotopoulou, A. & O'Riordan, K. (2017). Training to self-care: Fitness tracking, biopedagogy and the healthy consumer. *Health Sociology Review*, 26(1), 54–68.

Fox, S. & Duggan, M. (2013). Tracking for health. Retrieved 13 August 2016 from www.pewinternet.org/2013/01/28/tracking-for-health/.

Francombe, J. (2010). 'I cheer, you cheer, we cheer': Physical technologies and the normalized body. *Television & New Media*, 11(5), 350–366.

Francombe-Webb, J. (2016). Critically encountering exer-games and young femininity. *Television & New Media*, 17(5), 449–464.

Gardner, P. & Jenkins, B. (2016). Bodily intra-actions with biometric devices. *Body & Society*, 22(1), 3–30.

Ghaznavi, J. & Taylor, L.D. (2015). Bones, body parts, and sex appeal: An analysis of #thinspiration images on popular social media. *Body Image*, 14, 54–61.

Gorm, N. & Shklovski, I. (2016). Sharing steps in the workplace: Changing privacy concerns over time. *CHI '16 Proceedings of the 2016 CHI Conference on Human Factors in Computing Systems*, 4315–4319.

Hall, S. (1993). Encoding, decoding. In S. During (Ed.), *The cultural studies reader* (pp. 90–103). London: Routledge.

Hamari, J. & Koivisto, J. (2015a). 'Working out for likes': An empirical study on social influence in exercise gamification. *Computers in Human Behavior*, 50, 333–347.

Hamari, J. & Koivisto, J. (2015b). Why do people use gamification services? *International Journal of Information Management*, 35(4), 419–431.

Hartley, J. (1992). *Tele-ology: Studies in television*. London: Routledge.

Higgs, P. & Gilleard, C. (2010). Generational conflict, consumption and the ageing welfare state in the United Kingdom. *Ageing & Society*, 30(8), 1439–1451.

Krebs, P. & Duncan, D.T. (2015). Health app use among US mobile phone owners: A national survey. *JMIR mHealth and uHealth*, *3*(4). DOI: 10.2196/mhealth.4924.

Lee, H.E. & Cho, J. (2016 [Online First]). What motivates users to continue using diet and fitness apps? Application of the uses and gratifications approach. *Health Communication*. DOI: 10.1080/10410236.2016.116799.

Lewallen, J. & Behm-Morawitz, E. (2016). Pinterest or thinterest? Social comparison and body image on social media. *Social Media + Society*, *2*(1). DOI: 10.1177/2056305116640559.

Livingstone, S. (2003). The changing nature and uses of media literacy. In R. Gill, A. Pratt, T. Rantanen & N. Couldry (Eds.), *Media@LSE electronic working papers, Volume 4*. London: London School of Economics and Political Science.

Lydecker, J.A., Cotter, E.W., Palmberg, A.A., Simpson, C.S., Kwitowski, M., White, K. & Mazzeo, S.E. (2016). Does this Tweet make me look fat? A content analysis of weight stigma on Twitter. *Eating and Weight Disorders – Studies on Anorexia, Bulimia and Obesity*, *21*(2), 229–235.

Meckbach, J., Gibbs, B., Almqvist, J. & Quennerstedt, M. (2014). Wii teach movement qualities in physical education. *Sport Science Review*, *23*(5–6), 241–266.

Millington, B. (2015). Exergaming in retirement centres and the integration of media and physical literacies. *Journal of Aging Studies*, *35*, 160–168.

Millington, B. & Wilson, B. (2010). Media consumption and the contexts of physical culture: Methodological reflections on a 'Third Generation' study of media audiences. *Sociology of Sport Journal*, *27*(1), 20–53.

Nafus, D. & Sherman, J. (2014). This one does not go up to 11: The quantified self movement as an alternative Big Data practice. *International Journal of Communication*, *8*, 1784–1794.

Nansen, B., Vetere, F., Robertson, T., Downs, J., Brereton, M. & Durick, J. (2014). Reciprocal habituation: A study of older people and the Kinect. *ACM Transactions on Computer-Human Interaction*, *21*(3). DOI: http://dx.doi.org/10.1145/2617573.

The Nielsen Company. (2016). Hacking health: How consumers use smartphones and wearable tech to track their health. Retrieved 18 August 2016 from www.nielsen.com/us/en/insights/news/2014/hacking-health-how-consumers-use-smartphones-and-wearable-tech-to-track-their-health.html.

Rooksby, J., Rost, M., Morrison, A. & Chalmers, M. (2014). Personal tracking as lived informatics. *CHI '14 Proceedings of the SIGCHI Conference on Human Factors in Computing Systems*, 1163–1172.

Ruckenstein, M. (2014). Visualized and interacted life: Personal analytics and engagements with data doubles. *Societies*, *4*(1), 68–84.

Ruckenstein, M. & Pantzar, M. (2017). Beyond the quantified self: Thematic exploration of a dataistic paradigm. *New Media & Society*, *19*(3), 401–418.

Simpson, C.C. & Mazzeo, S.E. (2017). Skinny is not enough: A content analysis of fitspiration on Pinterest. *Health Communication*, *32*(5), 560–567.

Smith, G.J.D. & Vonthethoff, B. (2017). Health by numbers? Exploring the practice and experience of datafied health. *Health Sociology Review*, *26*(1), 6–21.

So, J., Prestin, A., Lee, L., Wang, Y., Yen, J. & Chou, W.-Y.S. (2015). What do people like to 'share' about obesity? A content analysis of frequent retweets about obesity on Twitter. *Health Communication*, *31*(2), 193–206.

Song, H., Peng, W. & Lee, K.M. (2011). Promoting exercise self-efficacy with an exergame. *Journal of Health Communication*, *16*(2), 148–162.

Szto, C. & Gray, S. (2015). Forgive me Father for I have thinned: Surveilling the bio-citizen through Twitter. *Qualitative Research in Sport, Exercise and Health*, 7(3), 321–337.

Tiggemann, M. & Zaccardo, M. (2015). 'Exercise to be fit, not skinny': The effect of fitspiration imagery on women's body image. *Body Image*, 15, 61–67.

Tremblay, M.S. & Lloyd, M. (2010). Physical literacy measurement: The missing piece. *Physical and Health Education Journal*, 76(1), 26–30.

Van Dijck, J. (2014). Datafication, dataism and dataveillance: Big data between scientific paradigm and ideology. *Surveillance & Society*, 12(2), 197–208.

Vickey, T.A., Ginis, K.M. & Dabrowski, M. (2013). Twitter classification model: The ABC of two million fitness tweets. *Translational Behavioral Medicine*, 3(3), 304–311.

White, N.J. (2007). Seniors trade walkers for Wii. Retrieved 18 August 2016 from www.thestar.com/life/2007/10/17/seniors_trade_walkers_for_wii.html.

Whitehead, M. (2001). The concept of physical literacy. *European Journal of Physical Education*, 6(2), 127–138.

Whitson, J.R. (2015). Foucault's Fitbit: Governance and gamification. In S. Walz & S. Deterding (Eds.), *The gameful world: Approaches, issues, applications* (pp. 339–358). Boston: MIT Press.

Wright, J. & Harwood, V. (2009). Biopower, biopedagogies and the obesity epidemic. In J. Wright & V. Harwood (Eds.), *Biopolitics and the 'obesity epidemic': Governing bodies* (pp. 1–14). New York: Routledge.

Conclusion

Amusing ourselves to life

"The American population is fat." Such is the opening broadside from Stephen Purpura et al. (2011) in their description of the technological system Fit4Life (p. 423). Designed on the basis of established principles in the persuasive technology literature, Fit4Life integrates wearable hardware and application software in the interest of promoting behavioural change in the areas of diet and exercise.

The system is robust. The Fit4Life Heart Rate Monitor is worn on the chest as an exercise-tracking tool. The Thinsert slides into one's shoe or sock and subsequently serves as a portable weighing device. The Earpiece – wearable too, of course – communicates verbally with the user and employs a Bluetooth receiver to connect with other parts of the system. It gets more complicated from there. For example, the Metabolic Lancet extracts blood from the toe at regular intervals so as to determine one's metabolic rate. Persuasion arises in one scenario described by Purpura et al. (2011) when Fit4Life attempts, rather bluntly, to direct the user's diet. "I'm sorry, Dave," a Fit4Life user is told, "you shouldn't eat that." Fit4Life continues, "Dave, you know I don't like it when you eat donuts." (p. 426). This is a fitting technological system for the new fitness boom.

Except that it's a hoax.

To be specific, Purpura et al. (2011) (eventually) reveal Fit4Life to be a fictional, critical design, the purpose being to show how computing systems can easily "spiral out of control" (p. 427), even if emerging from good intentions. The features of Fit4Life might seem extreme in their own right (drawing blood from the toe!) and might seem especially so when considered altogether. But the system logically extends principles of technology-mediated persuasion. In the process, the authors say, it raises critical issues related to both wearable technology and the pursuit of fit living – for example, over who has and should have control over defining health and fitness, over what the authors deem a troublesome trend towards self-optimization, and over the prominent role of surveillance and quantification in establishing truths of the self and manipulating behaviour. By bringing these issues to light, a key aim for Purpura et al. (2011) is to urge technology designers to think critically about their work. This is both a thought experiment and a practical intervention.

*****

What has become of fitness? As said in the introduction chapter of this book, in one sense, fitness is booming at the current moment in that, for some at least, business is booming. That Google, Apple, Microsoft, Sony, Facebook, Nintendo, Nike, adidas, and Reebok are now players in the fitness-technology 'complex' is perhaps the most significant indicator of fitness's perceived importance. Important too, however, is what fitness has come to *mean* through technological innovation. It was said at the outset of this book that fitness technologies are helping to fundamentally transform what is possible through fitness activity. Let us assess, then, the apparent traits of the new fitness boom, or Fitness 2.0, by reflecting on the analyses presented in preceding chapters of this book.

Eight characteristics of the new fitness boom are presented in this final, concluding chapter. The new fitness boom, it is argued, is 1) socio-technical, 2) interactive, 3) data intensive, 4) mobile, 5) networked, 6) gamified, 7) individualized, and 8) commodified in ways both 'old' and 'new'. To be sure, identifying characteristics of fitness technologies in this way is not a definitive exercise. The state of the art of technology will continue to evolve; it is complex enough already that some facets of the fitness-technology landscape surely escape this analysis. But charting characteristics of the new fitness boom helps in understanding i) the present state of fitness technologies, ii) points of continuity and disruption with the past, and iii) where fitness in general, and fitness technologies in particular might well be headed in the future. Indeed, after outlining these eight characteristics in detail, this final chapter turns to a discussion of the significance of the fitness technologies described throughout this book and an assessment of their attendant problems. This discussion is informed by the theoretical traditions reviewed in the book's introductory chapter. Consideration is given to what might be done – an admittedly vexing question – in the face of a new fitness boom that shows no sign of ceding momentum.

The new fitness boom

The new fitness boom is 1) socio-technical

"We are never faced with objects or social relations," writes Bruno Latour (1990). "We are faced with chains which are associations of humans (H) and non-humans (NH)" (p. 110). Latour (1990) continues:

> So instead of asking 'is this social', 'is this technical or scientific', or asking 'are these techniques influenced by society' or is this 'social relation

influenced by techniques' we simply ask: has a human replaced a non-human? has a non-human replaced a human? has the competence of this actor been modified? has this actor – human or non-human – been replaced by another one? has the chain of association been extended or modified?

(p. 110)

The socio-technical dimension of the new fitness boom appears most clearly with the discursive positioning of fitness technologies as coaches and trainers. This is the delegation of typically human responsibilities to increasingly sophisticated non-humans. As seen in Chapter 3, for example, the shoe-attachable ambiorun 'pod' device assesses running form through a coaching algorithm. 'H' becomes 'NH': whereas a human coach might once have observed one's running technique in the interest of relaying advice – lengthen your stride! – the job can now purportedly be done by a wearable and portable coach that operates through the integrated capacities of the shoe-attachable pod (hardware) and the smartphone-compatible ambiorun app (software).

In consumption, then, things are made out to be just like people. Equally, people are urged to come together with things to modify their competencies for the sake of optimization. Here it would be a mistake to presume that fitness participants are discrete and strictly human entities before using, say, a Fitbit brand wearable device. A key theme of Chapter 1 is that the conflation of bodies and technologies in the fitness realm is historically engrained. The ancient Greeks coated themselves with substances like clay and terracotta for physiological purposes. In the time of the physical culture movement, the strongman Eugen Sandow implored consumers to strap into his leg machine, replete as it was with hung stirrups (for the feet) connected to elastic cables. In the first fitness boom, devices like the Lifecycle 6500HR, an upright bike, assessed the body through technologies such as handlebar-embedded heart rate monitors. Nintendo's claim that, with the Wii Remote in hand, you *are* the controller, is perhaps the clearest articulation of how, in the new fitness boom, people are mechanized just as much as technologies are anthropomorphized. But people and things were already intertwined.

Moreover, non-humans themselves emerge from somewhere – which is to say, from chains of association that manifest in production. One of the lessons of Nintendo's adoption of fitness motifs, as described in Chapter 2, is that fitness technologies spring from the combined agencies of humans and constituent non-humans alike. Sensor technology provides a case in point on the non-human side of things. Humans join the fray as sport scientists, data scientists, engineers, venture capitalists, and manual labourers at Foxconn facilities, among many others. Again, it would be wrong to presume that in production, either humans or non-humans are independent and bounded entities. The Wii Fit Balance Board – ready in consumption to merge with the body – was built when Nintendo developers appropriated an optical rotary encoder from the controller of a previous Nintendo console (see Chapter 2). In this case, the competence of the Balance Board was modified through a chain of human and non-human associations as Nintendo producers worked with older, constituent parts. The outcome was that the Balance Board could measure the body within 100g of precision.

The new fitness boom is 2) interactive and 3) data intensive

This is a key theme of Chapter 3 especially. The point is that fitness technologies, through their embedded functionalities, help facilitate reciprocal relationships between people and their fitness technologies. In turn, and in the style of the big data movement writ large, data of potentially great variety can be generated in great volume.

This is a process that begins from the connection of flesh and technology at the point of the wrist and hand, the face and head, the legs and feet, the torso – anywhere, basically, where fitness merchants can fit their products. This is a haptic relationship that begets a form of haptic surveillance. The body and one's daily activities are codified through "metrics that matter" (Garmin Ltd., 2016) such as step count, distance or elevation travelled, BMI, body fat percentage, muscle mass, blood pressure variation, individual anaerobic threshold, and countless more. Important in this regard is the role played by algorithmic technology. The potential of sensor-generated raw data – that oxymoronic term (Gitelman & Jackson, 2013), given that sensors themselves are calibrated in production – would be unrealized if not converted through algorithms into intelligible metrics.

But this potential would go unrealized as well if data were not conveyed to consumers. Haptic surveillance begets self-surveillance through the integrated capacities of various technologies. A wristband communicates via Bluetooth to an app-loaded smartphone or tablet. And so the user has privy to data – both varied and voluminous – and to features like graphs showing changes in exercise performance or bodily composition over time. As said in Chapter 3, Wahoo Fitness promises to capture every "stride, crank, and squat" through its ecosystem of products – heart rate monitors, cycling sensors, apps of various kinds, and so on (Wahoo Fitness, 2016). From there, representing data is deemed a pathway to making exercise experience meaningful. If it's counted, it counts.

Haptic surveillance and self-surveillance are thus two components of the 'surveillant assemblage' that lies at the core of the new fitness boom – which is to say, the collection of surveillance modalities brought together through the ostensibly desirable end of optimizing daily life (see Haggerty & Ericson, 2000). Moreover, haptic surveillance in particular is crucial to rendering fitness a matter of *prosumption* in the sense that fitness consumers do not just use technologies but engage in data production. Prosumption is not new to fitness, but is newly intensified as data are generated *automatically* and *passively* as users go about their days, wearable devices in tow. In the idealized version of events, producing data inspires new insight and potentially behaviour change as well. Data production continues anew, and so the cycle of interactivity goes on.

The new fitness boom is 4) mobile and 5) networked

Mobility was the main theme of Chapter 4 of this book. The data intensive nature of the new fitness boom arises in one sense out of the sophistication of fitness technologies in capturing movement patterns or in taking snapshots of bodily composition. But it also follows from the 'anywhere', 'anytime' logic that now characterizes the experience of fitness tracking.

The questions explored in Chapter 4 pertain first to the factors that facilitate our seemingly frictionless fitness landscape. Portability is, of course, a first factor. Once fitness technologies are made compatible with portable devices or are made wearable in their own right, the spatial constraints on monitoring fitness activity grow ever less important. Fashionability and functionality are important precursors to mobility as well. For the former, 'anywhere' and 'anytime' fitness tracking is hardly possible if spaces such as the corporate boardroom are off limits for such purposes; hence, the fusion of fitness and fashion through the making of (for example) fitness tracking jewellery. Functionality is important in that fitness technologies are not just portable but are allegedly effective in a wide range of contexts. Sleep tracking, for example, is crucial to the idea that products like wrist-worn tracking devices fulfil a 24/7 service.

Convergence is a final factor in enabling mobility – convergence in the sense of compatibility across technological platforms. Perhaps most compelling in this regard is the development of 'open ecosystems' such as Google Fit that house data collected across a range of health and fitness platforms (e.g., a wearable tracker, a diet tracking app, and a sleep tracking device). The benefit of this arrangement is that consumers can make use of specialty hardware and software in generating data while at the same time storing their results in one place for the sake of simplicity. Open-source APIs are aimed at inspiring entrepreneurs to develop apps that work with overarching platforms like Google Fit, providing further options for fitness-inclined consumers.

From a cultural studies perspective, the mobile nature of the new fitness boom reflects the evolution of mobile privatization, a concept first developed by Raymond Williams (2004 [1974]). A mobile and private life once meant buying technologies of various kinds – workout equipment included, perhaps – as part of a physical move away from urban spaces that served as hubs for production and political activity. Mobile privatization is wrenchingly extended (Schiller, 2007) as our technologies – again, fitness technologies included – travel with us anywhere and anytime. Mobility in this arrangement is both a material and immaterial construct. An app like Zombies, Run! (ZR) implores its users to move across outdoor terrain and to track themselves in the process. As Emma Witkowski (2015) argues, this can inspire new understandings of the physical landscapes that surround us. Equally, *data* are spreadable across platforms, and with systems like Google Fit are even spreadable across proprietary virtual spaces. This gives life to that old axiom that information wants to be free.

But mobile privatization has also meant staying in touch without literally being in touch (Tomlinson, 2007; also see Hutchins, 2011). TV and radio helped rationalize suburbanization in that one could stay connected to political and productive centres of society, even from afar. This is where the networked element of contemporary forms of fitness engagement explored in Chapter 3 becomes relevant. Specifically, fitness experience is depicted along the lines of what Lee Rainie and Barry Wellman (2012) call networked individualism. Communities are 'out there' to help instruct and inspire fitness participation; it is just down to our own flexible autonomy to find them and make the most of them. 'Accountability 2.0' is the language used in promotional materials for the app Lose It!: "In-person meetings are so last century" (FitNow Inc., 2016). Thus, fitness-technology merchants still promise inter-personal relationships, only now these relationships manifest along new, technologically mediated chains of association. Networking, like self-tracking, purportedly transcends space and time.

The new fitness boom is 6) gamified

This is the 'amusing' side of *Amusing Ourselves to Life*. Chapter 3 explored the gamified dimension of the new fitness boom, with gamification understood as the application of game-design elements in non-gaming contexts. Gamification emerged out of the world of video gaming, and so it makes sense that Nintendo's fitness offerings feature the lure of gamification principles. But gamification is now relevant to fitness beyond the features of exergames like Wii Fit as well.

The app Fitocracy is an apt case in point in this regard in that it was built on the idea that fitness and fun need not be opposing forces (Fitocracy Inc., n.d.). The gamifying of Fitocracy instead is aimed at making fitness addictive through features like awarding badges for physical activity accomplishments and presenting them on an achievements dashboard. Fitocracy is not nearly alone in this regard. The tracking app RunKeeper, for example, has a leaderboard feature that can be synced with the user's existing online social networks (e.g., on Facebook). The leaderboard orders friends by activities completed: first place earns a ribbon next to her name to recognize her position; less active users – couch potatoes? – can earn a sofa icon instead (Miller, Cafazzo, & Seto, 2014; also see Lister et al., 2014).

For some critics, the problem of gamification is that it turns an end into a means. As Ian Bogost (2015) argues, gamification is "bullshit" in part in that it takes "playful experiences meant to produce gratification" and renders them "contorted techniques for producing compliance" (p. 72). The rejoinder here might well be that compliance is needed in the face of a pressing obesity epidemic and inactivity crisis. Based on results from a questionnaire administered to 200 Fitocracy users, Juho Hamari and Jonna Koivisto (2015a) found that the social features of the Fitocracy service had a positive relationship with i) use of Fitocracy, ii) exercise continuance, and iii) intention to recommend the technology to others (also see Hamari & Koivisto, 2015b). Still, the point remains: gamification in the new fitness boom helps rationalize an approach to health and fitness based on radically quantifying lived experience through commodity engagement. This is not just a matter of compliance, but compliance to fitness in a particular form.

The new fitness boom is 7) individualized

The individualizing of fitness-technology experience is implicit in several of the points made earlier. Self-surveillance is nothing if not an individualized pursuit. Mobility arises in the first instance in that fitness devices are both portable and personally owned. Even the communitarian dimensions of the new fitness boom are individualized in the sense that they often take the form of Accountability 2.0.

But a discourse of individualization arises in other ways as well. In one sense, the 'for everyone' discourse, as explored in Chapters 2 and 3, is relevant in this regard: fitness technologies are allegedly for everyone in that everyone is a potential consumer. This was Nintendo's gambit in developing the user-friendly Wii console and in placing health and fitness at the core of its product catalogue. For Fitbit, fitness technologies are for everyone in that Fitbit brand product offerings run the gamut from those aimed at beginners to those for attracting experts.

In another sense, fitness technologies are for everyone in that self-optimization evidently knows no bounds. As said in Chapter 3, optimization operates through the twin logics of susceptibility and enhancement. Susceptibility involves identifying and treating even asymptomatic problems. As an anthropomorphic coach, ambiorun can guide your running style and training intensity in the interest of steering you away from injury-inducing – which is to say, risky – habits (ambiorun UG, n.d.). The weight-to-height measure BMI is inherently a statement on susceptibility in that it categorizes people as underweight, normal, overweight, or obese. Enhancement, the other arm of optimization, means improving "almost any capacity of the human body or soul" (Rose, 2007, p. 82). Performance in relation to specific metrics might always be improved. What is the upper limit on steps per day? But optimization pertains especially to the grander achievements allegedly made possible through engagement with fitness devices: empower yourself; be unstoppable; flourish; achieve more; be your best self; optimize your life – the list goes on. The 'for everyone' discourse, then, works in two ways: there's a fitness device for all of us as we peruse the fitness market; fitness devices provide personalized guidance *after* purchase as well.

Yet optimization is to an extent marketing fodder. What of people's actual experiences? What Chapter 5 showed in part is that fitness-technology experience tends to be filtered through the prism of wider personal experience, at least insofar as we can judge from existing research. People use devices like wrist-worn fitness trackers for a whole host of reasons. In directive tracking, for example, people work towards a particular goal. Fetishized tracking involves tracking for tracking's sake (Rooksby et al., 2014). Engaging with fitness technologies can also require the deft synchronization of media and physical literacies. In games like Wii Bowling, one must read what's on screen while at the same time moving the body properly. Failure in one realm affects the other. But perhaps the most significant point in considering consumer experiences in the new fitness boom involves people's capacity to engage in what Paula Gardner and Barbara Jenkins (2016) call 'affective labour'. Participants in Gardner and Jenkins's (2016) research deliberated, or tarried, with memory, experience, and pleasurable forms of embodiment as they engaged with data generated from electroencephalogram (EEG) and electrocardiogram (ECG) technologies. Data were processed through personal and *felt* experience. While fitness technologies thus demonstrate, in the first instance, the untenability of the nature/culture divide through features like haptic surveillance, the process of tarrying with memory undermines a second binary as *objective* data and *subjective* experience combine.

The new fitness boom is 8) commodified

In particular, it is commodified in ways both old and new. A fitness apparel company in the 1980s built value out of its own production and sales processes: shoes were made and sold, ideally for a profit. Commodification in the 'old' or traditional style involves the recent proliferation of purchasable fitness goods and services. As seen in Chapter 2, we are at the point where fitness companies are now de facto technology companies (witness Nike's activity-tracking wristband); technology companies for their part are quite naturally at home in the fitness realm (witness Google Fit). The upshot of the fitness-technology 'complex' is that consumers with adequate spending power have more options for getting fit than ever before.

At the same time, however, the commodification of fitness takes on a new form as surplus value is generated from the commercial expropriation of consumer-produced data. As Christopher Till (2014) writes, for technology users, the transformation of exercise into digital data might be regarded as a formative activity in understanding the self. Till (2014) continues, "For corporations who are compiling these data, however, by transforming heterogeneous exercise activities into a standardized, quantified form, they are able to be made into a valuable resource; data that can be sold to advertisers" (p. 458).

The commodification of consumer data shines new light on many of the points made earlier. The data intensive nature of fitness-technology experience makes sense in a context where consumer data is potentially a profit source. Mobility, meanwhile, should not so easily be taken for granted. The seemingly frictionless data landscape is perhaps not quite what it appears, as data are certainly not directionless. There is value in ensuring data flow towards enclosed and controlled proprietary spaces. Said otherwise, corporate *dataveillance* – meaning the systematic use of personal data for commercial purposes – is part of the surveillant assemblage of the new fitness boom as well (see Chapter 4). Gamification and optimization also take on a new dimension with the commodification of fitness in mind. If fitness is fun, and if, as Zygmunt Bauman (2011) says, it knows no upper limit, there is always reason to keep producing data. If data are literally valuable there is a political economic basis for this as well. The old axiom is inverted: information wants to be paid for (Anderson & Wolff, 2010). Moreover, a third binary is shown to be faulty. People produce both data and surplus value: labour invades leisure.

Amusing ourselves to life

A century ago, Bernarr Macfadden (1915), icon of physical culture, outlined a daily regimen for achieving 'vitality supreme':

> Rise from six to eight o'clock. Drink a cup of hot or cold water immediately upon rising.
> Take the thyroid-stimulating exercises. Followed by the spine-strengthening movements in combination with the hot-water-drinking. . . .
> Before breakfast indulge in a good laugh or a good little singing.
> Eat a light breakfast. . . .
> Throughout the day while following your daily duties remember the suggestions in reference to proper position. Make a continuous and never-ending fight to keep a straight spine. . . .
> Eat your first hearty meal between twelve and two o'clock. . . . Masticate thoroughly. . . .
> Try to take a walk some time during the day. Remember during this walk to practice the thyroid-stimulating exercise. . . .
> Some time during the day, if possible, take some form of outdoor exercise. . . .
> Try to get a good laugh or do a little singing before your evening meal. . . .
> During the evening, if convenient, take an air bath. . . .

> Retire early enough to awake thoroughly refreshed at proper rising time without the warning of an alarm clock.
>
> (p. 257–259)

By Macfadden's (1915) account, life was more onerous without vitality than with it. The trick was evidently to pursue vitality everywhere and always. Macfadden's was a *daily* regimen and one that implicated everything from chewing to breathing to exercise to sleep. Moreover, vitality was both a choice and an obligation. For men, the duty was to be "strong and splendid." For women, it was to be "healthy and perfect" (Macfadden, 1915, p. 3).

The new fitness boom is not a fitness revolution. Yes, it capitalizes on and helps push forward a string of computing revolutions – the transition from analogue to digital technology, the arrival of Web 2.0, and the development and proliferation of sensor technology among them. But the fitness boom directs technology towards that time-tested end: the conduct of conduct. This is a matter of governmentality. In particular, at the core of the new fitness boom lies a form of conducting conduct akin to Deleuze's (1992) conception of biopower in his description of post-disciplinary societies of control. The body is deconstructed and made intelligible through numerical passwords or codes, at times for the sake of risk assessment. In Deleuze's terms, individuals become 'dividuals'. Or, to quote Paul Rabinow (2005), people are understood as "a sum of diverse factors amenable to analysis by specialists" (p. 187) – it's just that the specialists in question are oftentimes anthropomorphized things. Moreover, fitness-technology engagement is a *continuous* matter. Institutional fitness spaces have not disappeared. But, as seen in Chapter 4, activity-tracking apps like Human proclaim to make the world and the gym coterminous. Thus, surveillance is both micro-targeted and spatially unconstrained. As Foucault (1977) writes in *Discipline & Punish*, disciplinary mechanisms have a tendency to become de-institutionalized: "to emerge from the closed fortresses in which they once functioned and to circulate in a 'free' state" (p. 211). Of course, for individuals-cum-dividuals, all of this is voluntary, at least in principle. Optimization and gamification are carrots more so than sticks – though the risk of burdening society in a time of an obesity epidemic and inactivity crisis makes for a health *imperative* as well.

Better yet, a *healthism* imperative is at play, with healthism understood as an ideology that locates responsibility for health at the level of the individual and as such does the work of neoliberalism in the realm of health in particular (Crawford, 1980, 2006). Perhaps no conceptual term is used with greater imprecision at present than neoliberalism (Bell & Green, 2016). The language of 'neoliberalization' might well be preferable in that it reminds us that neoliberalism is a particular force, one situated in contexts where (for example) public health systems still exist and are often still defended from privatization (see Ward & England, 2007). Even so, what we are dealing with in the new fitness boom are commercial solutions to personal problems – including problems to which we are susceptible but that *we might not even know exist* – through forms of intervention that act 'at a distance' from formal institutions, whether public or private. The marketplace presents an unimaginably long list of consumer options for getting fit and is buoyed in the process by regulatory frameworks that place wellness devices in their own, less regulated, category (see Chapter 4) and by flexible labour markets that place commodity production in low-cost enterprise zones (see Chapter 2). To be sure, the point from there is for technology users to embrace an ethic of posthumanism and attach themselves, quite literally, to technologies so as to in turn understand themselves in rather technical terms. But this is a decidedly liberal humanist enterprise as well, at least in how it is imagined in the promotion of fitness technologies. The point is to rationally and assiduously make oneself 'better' via commodity experience. It can well be said that self-care is a *moral* choice too. In a context where obesity is allegedly tantamount to a terrorist attack (see the introduction chapter) and where fat shaming proliferates online and offline both (see Chapter 5), the task of making the body a 'strong machine', as Macfadden (1915) once said, is not just a desirable thing but the right thing to do – a choice and a duty. Said otherwise, optimization necessarily has an inverse side. If some people are being their best selves through commodity engagement, the flip side is that, *by choice*, others are failing to do so. The rallying cry for Eugen Sandow in the time of the physical culture movement was rather blunt: weakness is a crime, don't be a criminal. The sentiment persists, but is now filtered through the optimistic marketing language of optimization.

What's more, self-care is a pretext for investment: it is a reason in the first instance for companies to search for new bodily sites for commodification and is subsequently a means for profit generation in that the body, once numerically reified, has value as well. The benefit of making fitness an always-on proposition is that it raises the spectre of having consumers turn themselves into producers of value – and in constant fashion to boot. Moreover, fitness functionalities have the further benefit of making technologies not designed exclusively for fitness make sense as consumer investments. Decades ago, Jane Fonda aptly observed that VCR hardware was crying out for software; exercise videos fulfilled a purpose beyond didactic fitness messaging. The entrée of the technology sector's biggest players into the fitness field is perfectly logical in that self-tracking, as a form of self-care, gives us (further) reason to stare constantly at our smartwatches, smartphones, and tablets.

In all, the relationship works in both ways. The new fitness boom advances the small-state neoliberal imperative by shifting responsibility for health "into the domain for which the individual is responsible and transforming it into a problem of 'self-care'" (Lemke, 2001, p. 201). At the same time, fitness technologies create value from what was once uncommodified. A run was once just a run; now it is potentially a source of surplus value production. We would do well to remember here that Bernarr Macfadden, while espousing the merits of bodily efficiency, was also an entrepreneur, selling resources like magazines and exercise apparatuses of various kinds. The new fitness boom is not a fitness revolution. It is the conduct of conduct conceived anew.

* * * * *

Has the relationship between computing systems and fitness 'spiralled out of control', as Purpura et al. (2011) warn in 'designing' Fit4Life? At the core of Neil Postman's (1986) critique of communication technology is the idea that the form of communication necessarily impacts its content (see the introduction chapter). Whereas written text and in-person dialogue generally lend themselves to exposition and nuance, television trades in the currency of sound bites and visual spectacles. We amuse ourselves to death as important things in life are presented through the same filter as trivial ones. The form of the new fitness boom, per the eight characteristics outlined earlier, is generally one of gamified self-assessment through personal, wearable, commercial technologies. The content involves highly personalized, generally quantified, shareable, and data intensive insights into the body and daily life.

To answer 'no' to the question at hand – to say that technologies have *not* spiralled out of control – is to accept the form and content of the new fitness boom. Such an answer might perhaps involve championing the logic of the marketplace. So long as people are buying fitness technologies – so long as consumers accept the form and content of the things they purchase – the marketplace is functioning properly. Consumers are speaking; industry is responding. From a different perspective, an answer of 'no' might involve pointing to the health-related threats that ostensibly imperil us – in particular, the obesity epidemic and related crisis of inactivity, as discussed in detail in this book's introductory chapter. Indeed, these two points of view can be brought together. Both public health organizations and the scientific literature on physical (in)activity are increasingly focused on *overall* energy expenditure as a key health concern, and not just energy output as it pertains to exercise 'proper' (e.g., see National Physical Activity Plan Alliance, 2016). The commercial promotion of health and fitness has long tracked against the state of knowledge in science and medicine (see Chapter 1). The idea that light-intensity activity – walking the stairs at work, for example – counts towards the pursuit of healthy living makes integrating health and fitness into both technology production and consumption a logical course of action. Fitness technologies are not spiralling out of control. They are demonstrating how technological entrepreneurialism can be bent towards solving health problems that are *themselves* spiralling in the wrong direction.

Yet the analysis presented in this book has given many reasons to be leery of the new fitness boom. There is the matter first of the labour conditions that undergird technology production. Reports of inhumane working conditions abound – inhumane not just in that they are at times dangerous, but in that, as Richard Maxwell and Toby Miller (2012) write, migrant workers are removed from family and friendship networks and lack access to "forms of cultural enjoyment and release" (p. 95). In this sense, the new fitness boom presses onward with the labour controversies that implicated companies like Nike in the time of the first fitness boom. To be fair, fitness does not so much cause but rather shines new light on the problem of manual labour in technology production. Engaging with family and friendship networks and partaking in forms of cultural enjoyment might well be regarded as part of an optimized daily routine.

There is the matter too of privacy and security. As said in Chapter 4, for example, a 2014 study by the GPEN found that 85% of the apps selected for GPEN's analysis – some of which were of the health and fitness variety – did not clearly explain their process of collecting, using, and disclosing personal information (see Office of the Privacy Commissioner of Canada, 2014). This, again, is a problem that extends far beyond the fitness realm. Every search engine query and social media post is now potentially subject to surveillance. But health and fitness data can of course be especially sensitive. The issue of hypocrisy is relevant in this case as well. As the Open Effect researchers (see Chapter 4) say based on their disconcerting assessment of privacy and security in a number of prominent wearable fitness technologies, "Can individuals be truly empowered when their data is not secured?" (Hilts, Parsons, & Knockel, 2016, p. 1).

A third issue: that, for consumers, fitness technologies might *hinder* as much as help in the pursuit of better living. To say optimization has an inverse side, as said earlier, is not just rhetoric. As shown in Chapter 5, the fact that commodity experience is actively negotiated is a double-edged sword. People make sense of ostensibly objective, and potentially objectifying, data by filtering them through personal and subjective experience. Yet our existing subject positions are always-already complex. As Hayeon Song, Wei Peng, and Kwan Min Lee (2011) found in studying the exergame *Eye-Toy: Kinect*, the game had a *negative* impact on people of high body image dissatisfaction, given that the imperfect self was set against an ideal standard presented on screen. Likewise, 'fitspiration' imagery on social media, while aimed at inspiring fitness engagement through the depiction of the body, lean and toned, has been shown to serve its purpose while *at the same time* heightening body dissatisfaction and hindering appearance self-esteem (Tiggemann & Zaccardo, 2015).

Fourth, and finally, to trade in the logic of personal empowerment is to overlook dimensions of health that exist far beyond the individual's control. Three decades ago, in the time of the first fitness boom, Alan Ingham (1985) offered a piercing criticism of the convergence of health promotion and lifestyle politics:

> What do we have to offer to the currently ill and the about-to-be-ill segments of the population; those whose illnesses have more to do with

workplace rather than lifestyle, with the ravages of unemployment rather than defects of character, with the cumulative effects of impoverishment – impoverishment which is becoming increasingly feminized? Shall we say that they should aerobicize, jazzercise, and jog their problems away? Shall we counsel them to internalize the locus of control?

(p. 54)

The social determinants of health pertain to matters such as social exclusion, unemployment, and lack of access to healthy food (Wilkinson & Marmot, 2003). Moreover, in the United Kingdom at least, the (neoliberal) politics of austerity have in recent years placed a downward pressure on local councils, in turn threatening closure for public leisure facilities (e.g., see Bingham, 2014; Conn, 2015; Findlay-King et al., 2017; Meegan et al., 2014; Parnell, Millward, & Spracklen, 2015). Shall we say under such conditions that people facing difficult circumstances should now track, share, and optimize their problems away? Shall we counsel them not only to internalize the locus of control but also to locate their problems in specific measures of the self? Instead of doing so, we might ask why we even need a new fitness boom. How is it that we are collectively in such a perilous position, having already gone through an initial fitness boom? Why will this new iteration work when the first fitness boom evidently didn't, if the twin crises of inactivity and obesity are any indication? The new fitness boom is not a fitness revolution. It takes the form of the first fitness boom and presses onward: fitness is *more* individualized, *more* interactive, and *more* commodified than ever before. Ingham (1985) continues, "If we continue in these, our present, practices, I doubt that we shall be saying much of substance, saying much that corresponds to experience with structural contradiction" (p. 54). It would seem that we have indeed 'continued in the present practices' of the mid-1980s – and that Ingham was right. Structural conditions are beyond the purview of the new fitness boom. The argument, in other words, is that fitness technologies do not just proffer but are *confined* to a flawed model of personal empowerment.

Amusing ourselves to life. No doubt it is an enticing proposition. The headless family watching TV (as best they can, one supposes) on the cover of Postman's (1986) book *Amusing Ourselves to Death* is a poor representation of contemporary technology experience. The family is spatially bound, sedentary, and, through the metaphor of decapitation, passive and unthinking. The analysis presented herein has shown present-day technology experience to be mobile, interactive, and negotiated. Even if we grant Postman leeway in recognizing that *Amusing Ourselves to Death* was written more than three decades ago – well before many of the technological advances described in previous chapters – his analysis, and the 'repressive' tradition of technology criticism in general, tends to overlook the productive dimensions of technological mediation in depicting technology experience as the negation of life.

But it would equally be a mistake to dismiss Postman out of hand. *Form and content*: the new fitness boom promises to make us healthier, yet the analysis presented in this book is suggestive of what happens when we subject health to a form of commercial intervention. Health is made personal. Health outcomes are made vague and spectacular. Health is unpicked from our local circumstances. Health data are ours, but probably not ours alone. When the logic of fitness is introduced into the mix – fitness being a construct, as Bauman (2011) says, with no upper limit – health can never actually be attained. Amusing ourselves to life is an enticing proposition indeed. But are fitness technologies spiralling out of control? At the very least, they are spiralling *away* from many of the things we know to be crucial to health.

Conclusion: the future of fit

It is surely a fool's errand to predict the future of technology development. The eight characteristics outlined earlier are valuable in highlighting historical trajectories, if not precise landing points. Perhaps most of all we should expect that, in a time of 'sensor mania' (Swan, 2012), tracking technology will continue to 'disappear' into the objects that surround us, the aim being to generate ever more data on daily life for sharing across technological platforms, and eventually for sharing with people too. The company iFit already imagines a healthy version of the 'Internet of Things' – for example, Internet-connected kitchen appliances that help deliver a personalized diet based on what they know from other technologies, such as an Internet-connected bed and a wearable tracking device (BusinessWire, 2015). Fit4Life, the faux technological system described at the outset of this chapter, appears not such an exaggerated design: Dave, you shouldn't eat that donut!

Tracking data is likely to continue branching in capillary-like fashion into new contexts as well, raising complicated ethical questions in the process. Tracker-generated data are already being used in court cases, for example. The agency of technology takes on a new dimension when a fitness tracker serves as a de facto expert witness. As Kate Crawford (2014) writes, questions abound. Will this change people's relationships with their wearable devices? Who is really testifying here? The device? Your body? An algorithm? If it's your body, is this self-incrimination? Questions worth adding: What to make of the fact that fitness trackers are differently calibrated, as seen in the introduction chapter, meaning one device might give different testimony from another? What to make of the security vulnerabilities of 'amusing' fitness technologies, given their growing role in very serious contexts of this kind?

The functionalities of fitness technologies are also likely to impact on health and fitness norms in the years ahead, though precisely how this will happen remains unclear. BMI, for example, is a rather crude metric. Might we see striations within the categories of 'underweight', 'normal', 'overweight', and 'obese'? Might we see a labelling system not only for the state of the body but also for one's typical daily activity level as well? Will people be labelled not just overweight but overweight/sedentary on the basis of purportedly objective assessments? Perhaps, by contrast, there is cause for optimism in that fitness data will help contest the idea that overweight and obesity are reducible to laziness or that they are necessarily correlated to poor health. Perhaps workers will show how inhumane labour conditions can be by producing and sharing objective data that demonstrate how long they stand on a daily basis. The future of fitness is unclear, though the characteristics outlined earlier are a starting point in considering what is to come in the years ahead.

Moreover, it is difficult to make recommendations for change with the current state of fitness technologies in mind. The new fitness boom is entangled with wider trends in such a way that solutions to the problems outlined earlier are to a great extent beyond the scope of this analysis. The problem of labour conditions in manual production, for instance, is one of holding powerful and often transnational companies to account – not just that, but of doing so in a time when the neoliberal argument on the merits of flexible labour and deregulation has become hegemonic. Likewise, the notion of 'responsibilizing' health at the level of the individual is now so socially engrained that it tacitly permeates even *criticism* of fitness technologies. To compare tracking devices X and Y in the task of counting steps is a worthwhile cause in that it can reveal the subjectiveness of purportedly objective data (see the introduction chapter). But the implication of research of this kind is arguably that we simply need to measure *better*. To paraphrase Evgeny Morozov's (2015) incisive critique of technology criticism itself, health – a social and political problem that might be dealt with at the level of citizens and institutions – becomes a technical problem to be dealt with at the level of production and consumption.

These are of course not reasons to give up the cause of social change entirely. A fascinating element of the new fitness boom is that it makes fitness into something that is not just for us, but *about us* (Crawford, Lingel, & Karppi, 2015; also see Bossewitch & Sinnreich, 2013; Van Dijck, 2009, 2013). In buying and selling, consumers become the thing that is bought and sold. This is disconcerting for reasons outlined earlier, but it can equally be used as a heuristic device in the pursuit of a more critically engaged future with fitness technologies. That is to say, we should welcome initiatives that turn an analytical lens on fitness technologies themselves: initiatives that are not *for* technologies, in the sense of deploying them as intended, but are *about technologies* in the sense of shining a critical light on how they work, and how they might be made both different and differently. Says Postman (1986): no technology is dangerous in the extreme so long as its dangers are well known. Our public institutions hold potential in this regard in particular. We should welcome, then, any school-based initiative that asks students to critically examine fitness technologies and their implications, and does not simply use technology in pursuit of fitness-related outcomes. We should welcome experiments from researchers that, in the style Gardner and Jenkins's (2016) research, have people engage with technology-generated data in hopes of understanding how data are processed on a personal level, as well as research that, in the style of GPEN's or Open Effect's analyses, critically probes into matters of privacy and security. We should welcome investigative reports on both manual and knowledge labour as they pertain to technologies – fitness technologies included. And we should welcome government attempts at understanding and debating how data are produced and exchanged and at regulating technology companies with consumer interests in mind. The Open Effect study was, after all, supported by the Canadian government. We should welcome, and, indeed, we should actively pursue such initiatives.

At the same time, we should welcome initiatives that aim to recognize what is *lost* given the form and content of contemporary fitness technologies. The idea that leisure facilities and public health care systems are unsustainable is not separate from, but rather is part and parcel of the logic that undergirds the new fitness boom. What is lost in the quest for personalized, market-based solutions to allegedly private problems is the idea that our local circumstances are not so easily transcended, that health is not reducible to personal choice, and that 'warm' in-the-flesh experts are still important – a human coach, after all, does more than proffer technical advice. What can be done is to recognize and fight for the sustained existence of that which the new fitness boom seemingly deems irrelevant.

If nothing else, the recommendation is this: lest we find ourselves headless, the prospect of amusing ourselves to life should be taken seriously indeed.

References

ambiorun UG. (n.d.). Retrieved 13 June 2016 from www.ambiorun.com/.

Anderson, C. & Wolff, M. (2010). The web is dead: Long live the internet. Retrieved 8 July 2016 from www.wired.com/magazine/2010/08/ff_webrip/.

Bauman, Z. (2011). *Liquid life*. Cambridge: Polity Press.

Bell, K. & Green, J. (2016). On the perils of invoking neoliberalism in public health critique. *Critical Public Health*, 26(3), 239–243.

Bingham, J. (2014). Parks and leisure centres under threat as ageing population swallows council budgets. Retrieved 20 April 2017 from www.telegraph.co.uk/news/health/elder/11189980/Parks-and-leisure-centres-under-threat-as-ageing-population-swallows-council-budgets.html.

Bogost, I. (2015). Why gamification is bullshit. In S. Walz & S. Deterding (Eds.), *The gameful world: Approaches, issues, applications* (pp. 65–79). Boston: MIT Press.

Bossewitch, J. & Sinnreich, A. (2013). The end of forgetting: Strategic agency beyond the panopticon. *New Media & Society*, 15(2), 224–242.

BusinessWire. (2015). The iFit life booth demonstrates a healthy 'Internet of Things' at #CES2015. Retrieved 21 April 2017 from www.businesswire.com/news/

home/20150106006669/en/iFit-Life-Booth-Demonstrates-Healthy-%E2%
80%9CInternet-Things%E2%80%9D.

Conn, D. (2015). Olympic legacy failure: Sports centres under assault by thousand council cuts. Retrieved 20 April 2018 from www.theguardian.com/sport/2015/jul/05/olympic-legacy-failure-sports-centres-council-cuts.

Crawford, K. (2014). When Fitbit is the expert witness. Retrieved 21 April 2017 from www.theatlantic.com/technology/archive/2014/11/when-fitbit-is-the-expert-witness/382936/.

Crawford, K., Lingel, J. & Karppi, T. (2015). Our metrics, ourselves: A hundred years of self-tracking from the weight scale to the wrist wearable device. *European Journal of Cultural Studies*, *18*(4–5), 479–496.

Crawford, R. (1980). Healthism and the medicalization of everyday life. *International Journal of Health Services*, *10*(3), 365–388.

Crawford, R. (2006). Health as a meaningful social practice. *Health*, *10*(4), 401–420.

Deleuze, G. (1992). Postscript on the societies of control. *October*, *59*, 3–7.

Findlay-King, L., Nichols, G., Forbes, D. & Macfadyen, G. (2017 [Online First]). Localism and the Big Society: The asset transfer of leisure centres and libraries – fighting closures or empowering communities? *Leisure Studies*.

FitNow Inc. (2016). How it works. Retrieved 13 June 2016 from www.loseit.com/how-it-works/.

Fitocracy Inc. (n.d.). About us. Retrieved 13 June 2016 from www.fitocracy.com/about-us/.

Foucault, M. (1977). *Discipline and punish: The birth of the prison*. New York: Pantheon Books.

Gardner, P. & Jenkins, B. (2016). Bodily intra-actions with biometric devices. *Body & Society*, *22*(1), 3–30.

Garmin Ltd. (2016). Vivo fitness. Retrieved 12 June 2016 from http://explore.garmin.com/en-GB/vivo-fitness/.

Gitelman, L. & Jackson, V. (2013). Introduction. In L. Gitelman (Ed.), *'Raw data' is an oxymoron* (pp. 1–14). Cambridge: MIT Press.

Haggerty, K.D. & Ericson, R.V. (2000). The surveillant assemblage. *British Journal of Sociology*, *51*(4), 605–622.

Hamari, J. & Koivisto, J. (2015a). 'Working out for likes': An empirical study on social influence in exercise gamification. *Computers in Human Behavior*, *50*, 333–347.

Hamari, J. & Koivisto, J. (2015b). Why do people use gamification services? *International Journal of Information Management*, *35*(4), 419–431.

Hilts, A., Parsons, C. & Knockel, J. (2016). Every step you fake: A comparative analysis of fitness tracker privacy and security (Open Effect Report). Retrieved 8 July 2016 from https://openeffect.ca/reports/Every_Step_You_Fake.pdf.

Hutchins, B. (2011). The acceleration of media sport culture. *Information, Communication & Society*, *14*(2), 237–257.

Ingham, A. (1985). From public issue to personal trouble: Well-being and the fiscal crisis of the state. *Sociology of Sport Journal*, *2*, 43–55.

Latour, B. (1990). Technology is society made durable. *The Sociological Review*, *38*(S1), 103–131.

Lemke, T. (2001). 'The birth of bio-politics': Michel Foucault's lecture at the Collège de France on neo-liberal governmentality. *Economy and Society*, *30*(2), 190–207.

Lister, C., West, J.H., Cannon, B., Sax, T. & Brodegard, D. (2014). Just a fad? Gamification in health and fitness apps. *JMIR Serious Games*, 2(2). DOI: http://doi.org/10.2196/games.3413.

Macfadden, B. (1915). *Vitality supreme*. New York City: Physical Culture Publishing Co.

Maxwell, R. & Miller, T. (2012). *Greening the media*. Oxford: Oxford University Press.

Meegan, R., Kennett, P., Jones, G. & Croft, J. (2014). Global economic crisis, austerity and neoliberal urban governance in England. *Cambridge Journal of Regions, Economy and Society*, 7(1), 137–153.

Miller, A.S., Cafazzo, J.A. & Seto, E.S. (2014). A game plan: Gamification design principles in mHealth applications for chronic disease management. *Health Informatics Journal*, 22(2), 184–193.

Morozov, E. (2015). The taming of tech criticism. *The Baffler*, 27. Retrieved 21 April 2017 from http://thebaffler.com/salvos/taming-tech-criticism.

National Physical Activity Plan Alliance. (2016). 2016 United States report card on physical activity for children and youth. Retrieved 28 April 2017 from www.physicalactivityplan.org/projects/reportcard.html.

Office of the Privacy Commissioner of Canada. (2014). News release: Global privacy sweep raises concerns about mobile apps. Retrieved 8 July 2016 from www.priv.gc.ca/en/opc-news/news-and-announcements/2014/nr-c_140910/.

Parnell, D., Millward, P. & Spracklen, K. (2015). Sport and austerity in the UK: An insight into Liverpool 2014. *Journal of Policy Research in Tourism, Leisure and Events*, 7(2), 200–203.

Postman, N. (1986). *Amusing ourselves to death: Public discourse in the age of show business*. New York: Penguin Books.

Purpura, S., Schwanda, V., Williams, K., Stubler, W. & Sengers, P. (2011). Fit4life: The design of a persuasive technology promoting healthy behavior and ideal weight. *CHI '14, Proceedings of the SIGCHI Conference on Human Factors in Computing Systems*, 423–432.

Rabinow, P. (2005). Artificiality and enlightenment: From sociobiology to biosociality. In J.X. Inda (Ed.), *Anthropologies of modernity: Foucault, governmentality, and life politics* (pp. 181–193). Oxford: Blackwell Publishing Ltd.

Rainie, L. & Wellman, B. (2012). *Networked: The new social operating system*. Cambridge: MIT Press.

Rooksby, J., Rost, M., Morrison, A. & Chalmers, M. (2014). Personal tracking as lived informatics. *CHI '14 Proceedings of the SIGCHI Conference on Human Factors in Computing Systems*, 1163–1172.

Rose, N. (2007). *The politics of life itself: Biomedicine, power, and subjectivity in the twenty-first century*. Princeton: Princeton University Press.

Schiller, D. (2007). *How to think about information*. Urbana: University of Illinois Press.

Song, H., Peng, W. & Lee, K.M. (2011). Promoting exercise self-efficacy with an exergame. *Journal of Health Communication*, 16(2), 148–162.

Swan, M. (2012). Sensor mania! The internet of things, wearable computing, objective metrics, and the quantified self 2.0. *Journal of Sensor and Actuator Networks*, 1(3), 217–253.

Tiggemann, M. & Zaccardo, M. (2015). 'Exercise to be fit, not skinny': The effect of fitspiration imagery on women's body image. *Body Image*, 15, 61–67.

Till, C. (2014). Exercise as labour: Quantified self and the transformation of exercise into labour. *Societies*, 4(3), 446–462.

Tomlinson, J. (2007). *The culture of speed: The coming of immediacy*. London: Sage.

Van Dijck, J. (2009). Users like you? Theorizing agency in user-generated content. *Media, Culture & Society*, 31(1), 41–58.

Van Dijck, J. (2013). *The culture of connectivity: A critical history of social media*. Oxford: Oxford University Press.

Wahoo Fitness. (2016). About us. Retrieved 13 June 2016 from http://uk.wahoofitness.com/about-us.

Ward, K. & England, K. (2007). Introduction: Reading neoliberalization. In K. England & K. Ward (Eds.), *Neoliberalization* (pp. 1–22). Hoboken: Blackwell.

Wilkinson, R.G. & Marmot, M. (2003). *Social determinants of health: The solid facts* (Second edition). Copenhagen: World Health Organization.

Williams, R. (2004 [1974]). *Television: Technology and cultural form*. London: Fontana.

Witkowski, E. (2015 [Online First]). Running with zombies: Capturing new worlds through movement and visibility practices with Zombies, Run! *Games and Culture*. DOI: 10.1177/1555412015613884.

Index